Easy Recipes for Hard Days

Shannon E. Gale

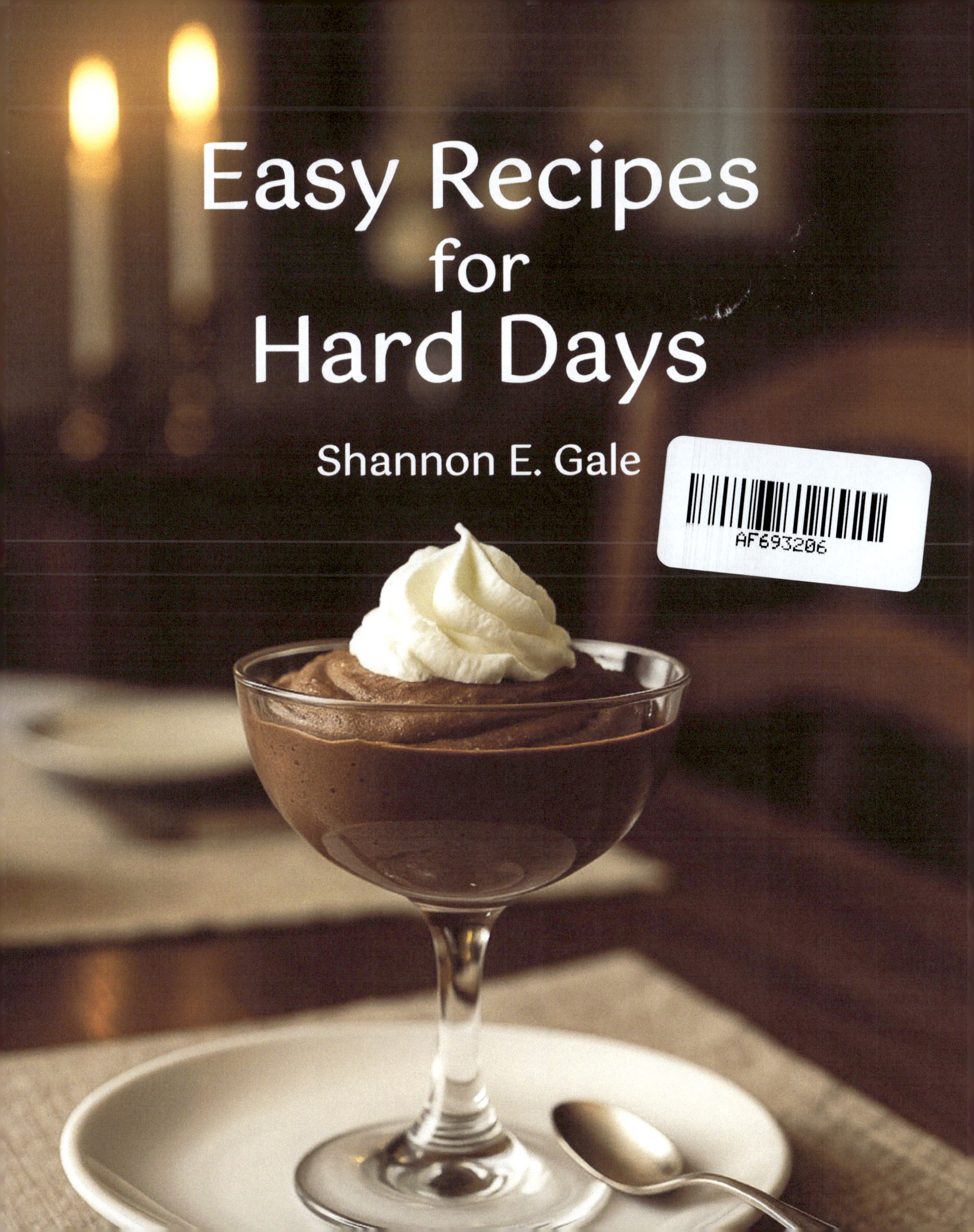

The Crisis Cookbook: Easy Recipes and Meal Planning for Homemade Nutrition When You Don't Feel Like Cooking

First Comes Love LLC
Frankfort, Kentucky, USA

ISBN paperback: 978-1-965020-03-6
ASIN ebook B0G2D3NPWQ:

All images were either photographed or generated with ChatGPT by Shannon E. Gale
All design and formatting of the cover and book interior were accomplished by Shannon E. Gale.

Dedication

To Brandon Gale, Edison Gale, Kathy Gale, Dr. Ashley Gale Smith, Kristin Heather Gale, Jason Smith, Joshu Goebeler, Paxton Smith, and Ajay Smith.

In loving memory of Dr. Steven H. Gale.

And to all people everywhere who are having a hard day.

Table of Contents

Acknowledgements

Thank you to everyone who replied to my posts on social media with suggestions and requests for how to structure this cookbook.

Thank you to those who provided me with beautiful ingredients and those who inspired some of the recipes in this book: Ayres Family Orchard, Brenneman and Bucks Farm (Cody Brenneman), Selina Britton, Melissa Calhoun, Cedar Ring Greens (Connie Lemley), Patrick Cichy, CommonWealth Gardens, John Downing, Evans Orchard, Eddie Fowler, Franklin County Farmers Market, Fritz's Apiary (Fritz and Shawchyi Vorisek), Brandon Gale, Linda Gale, Steven Gale, Colleen Gehlbach, Jessie Hancock, Happy Jacks Pumpkin Farm, Bob Hawes, Hazelfield Farm (Esmee McKee and Todd Elliott), Marcia Johnson, LM Sugarbush, Locals Food Hub, Mulberry Orchard, Hillary Nadeau, Rough Draft Farmstead (Jesse Frost and Hannah Crabtree), Beth Ruggles, and Amy Slack.

Thank you to my husband and son for being my live-in taste-testers and always helping to wash the dishes.

Thank you most of all to Kathy Gale for her editing services and cooking inspiration.

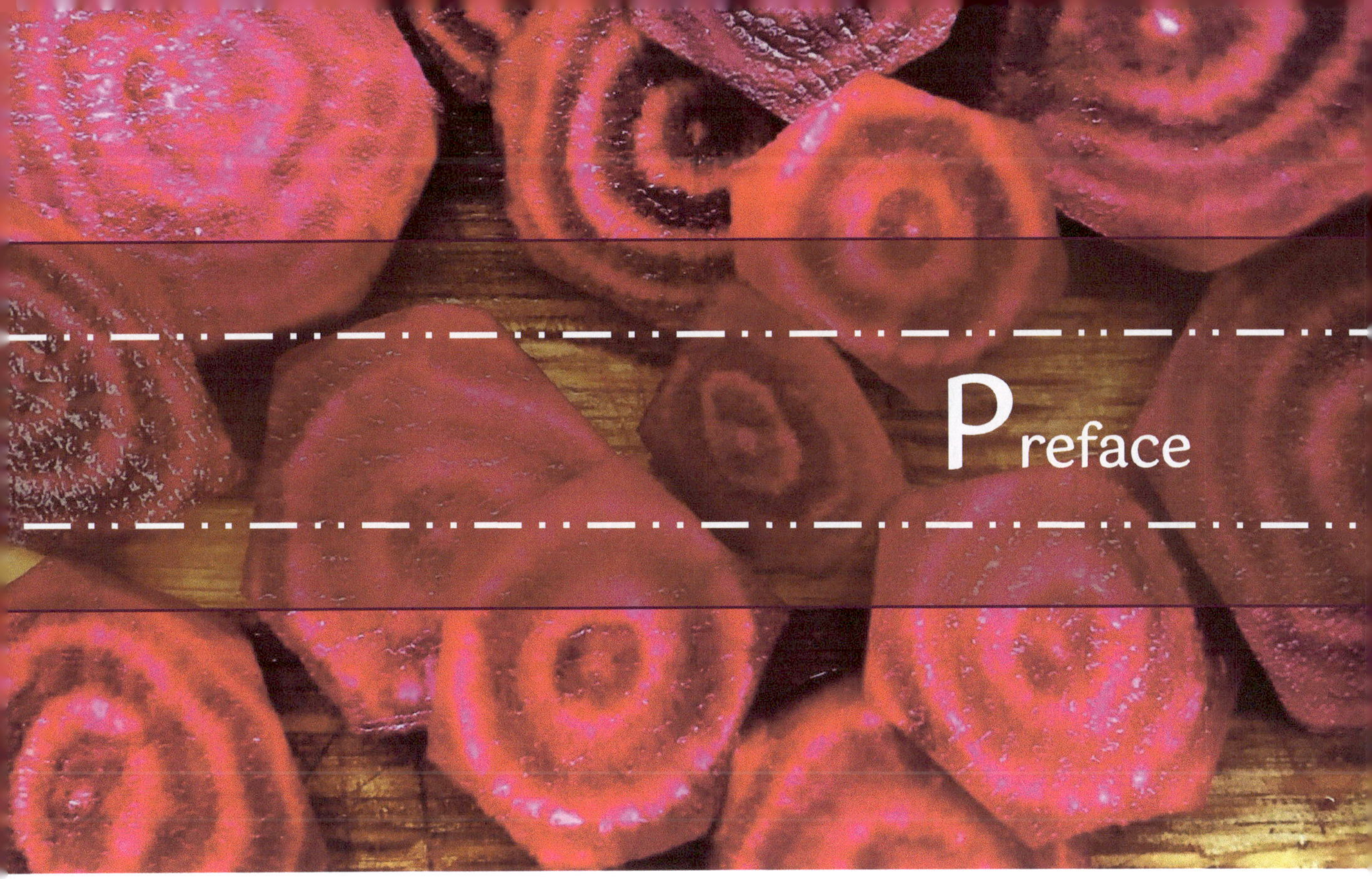

Preface

To Be Acquainted with Sadness

If you have picked up this cookbook, you are probably holding sadness or stress, or both, in your heart. You might be feeling a lot of pain, physical or emotional, or both. Life feels unmanageable, or the things that matter are out of grasp...probably both. Eating well is impossible.

It is hard to imagine that anything will ever get better. But these experiences come in seasons. Hard days are not the only kind you will ever know.

Seasons of crisis can make us feel very alone, but I assure you that many others have been through crises before you. They have survived and lived to tell the story. I am one of them.

Crisis Affects Our Appetite

I lived with a chronic illness for many years — at the same time as running 5 businesses and being a full-time, homeschooling, single mom. I have also moved to new homes, lost loved ones, experienced pregnancy and postpartum complications, and had my heart broken. I know what it is to be in crisis.

I tend to be an emotional starver: if I'm upset, I can't eat. I lose too much weight. When we have a lot to deal with, it makes sense for our bodies not to have to deal with digestion, too. But food is a necessity of life, and when we can find that one recipe that is palatable even when we don't want to eat – maybe it's even delicious – it can make all the difference in the world!

Every now and then, though, emotions have had me eating too much of the kinds of food that put on excessive weight. If our bodies think that famine and hardship are coming, they will take precautions to get through the future lean times. For the most part, though, the extra weight isn't actually necessary and leads to further health complications.

Health Concerns

It's known that, counterintuitive as it may be, hospital waiting room vending machines are filled with junk food. Crunchy, salty, and overly sweet foods are what we crave when we are worried, exhausted, and too busy for a real meal. Of course, these foods aren't good for anyone, but for those with a chronic illness, they can be even worse.

One of the most obnoxious health conditions that I have dealt with is Mast Cell Activation Syndrome (MCAS). This condition can make people unexpectedly sensitive to a lot of foods and chemicals. For some people, this can mean that a certain kind of chips is the only food they can always eat without getting sick. But for others, like me, the chemicals in most processed, prepackaged, and restaurant foods can cause awful symptoms.

Many other health conditions can flare up during times of stress, as well, so healthy eating is of paramount importance during crisis. Everyone finds healthy eating on hard days to be challenging, and it is only by the grace of God that I discovered easy recipes and strategies for eating well through times of grief, stress, and chronic illness.

Let Food Feed Your Soul

One of the ways in which I was graced with healthy eating was discovering that my small town was surrounded by organic and biodynamic farms producing vegetables, fruits, grains, dairy, meat, herbs, and eggs. Not only were the foods readily available, they were also inexpensive...and every item I cooked had been nurtured and respectfully harvested by someone who was a friend to me.

Sometimes, on days when my head hurt so much that I could barely open my eyes and my body was weak and shaky, I knew that the best thing for me would be some homemade food. I learned to cook easy meals, and as I prepared them, I found wells of gratitude in my heart.

The beets that I sliced revealed brilliant fuschia and pink patterns. The carrots were so crisp they split neatly beneath my knife. The apples hid five-pointed stars inside. The rainbow-hued berries needed no attention from me to be bite-sized and delightful.

I was blessed to be able to prepare fresh, homemade food with whole ingredients, love, reverence, and gratitude. I want to share that gift with you.

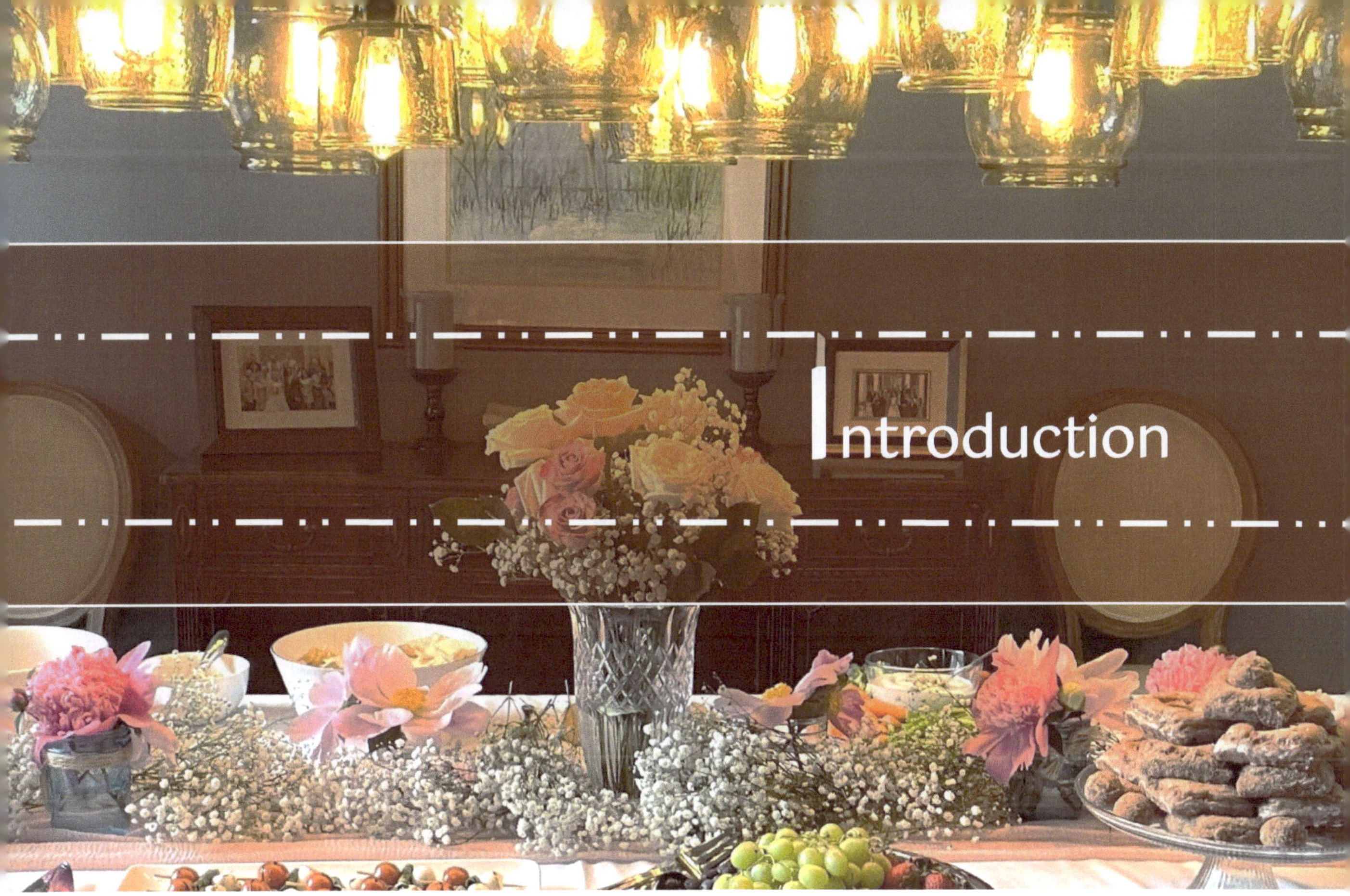

Introduction

You Deserve Good Food, Even Now

You may be going through something very difficult right now, and if you are, my heart goes out to you. I am praying for each person who reads this cookbook that you may feel peace and love, and that you may be comforted and strengthened by good food. You deserve it.

You deserve something better than the ultra-processed, poison-laden, anxiety-inducing, factory-packaged foods that most people eat when they don't have the ability to cook a homemade meal. (The synthetic ingredients in processed foods, such as dyes, preservatives, and artificial flavors, are made from petroleum, which is toxic to humans and causes numerous adverse health effects.)

Home cooking does not need to be difficult. Simplicity has been the way of home chefs for generations.

This book is for you if you are going through crisis, no matter what that crisis may be: illness, stress at work, heartbreak, moving to a new house, identity crisis, financial struggles. The human condition is sometimes one of struggle and suffering, but your need for wholesome food only increases in these times.

Feed yourself well, and you will walk through the struggles. You will eventually enter another phase of your life – one that is full of grace, ease, and contentment. Perhaps even joy.

And then, when you are thriving, you will have these nourishing recipes of comfort foods to prepare for friends and loved ones when they face their own struggles. The recipes are easy, so it will be a cinch for you to whip something up without sacrificing too much of your own time.

About the Recipes

All of the recipes in this book are favorites of my family – things I have prepared dozens and dozens of times.

They are generally intended for you to prepare for yourself as an individual. When you are in crisis, the last thing you need is more chopping or standing at the stove. There is no benefit to making more food than you can eat. If you are cooking for a family, these simple recipes are easily multiplied.

You will find that some recipes do make a larger portion; these are foods that freeze well in single-serving dishes and reheat easily.

These recipes are not finicky. Substitute anything you want! I cook with wheat flour, raw whole milk, and other foods that many people must or choose to avoid. Substitute with whatever your trusted ingredients may be. These recipes are not the kind of recipes that require careful measuring or specific ingredients. Be casual and cook what is best for you.

Join the Community

I'm so glad you're reading this book, and I hope that I can help you in many ways. I was inspired to put this cookbook together because I had written a book called *Hypermobile and Happy* about healing my chronic illness. Then, while I was getting the word out about holistic treatments for hypermobility-related conditions, I heard back from readers who were seeing improvement in their symptoms, but they still had some specific struggles...like figuring out how to cook with real ingredients while still struggling with chronic pain, fatigue, brain fog, joint instability, and dysautonomia. This cookbook is especially designed to help you along on your healing journey.

As I communicated with readers and raised awareness online, I got to know a lot of like-minded people on social media. We've become a supportive community, sharing ideas, lifting each other up through difficult times, and celebrating all the ways that our lives are getting better.

Use the QR code to find these communities online, or go to **www.shannonegale.com**. Follow me on Instagram, YouTube, LinkedIn, Substack, and Facebook. And be sure to join the facebook group **Holistic EDS, Hypermobile and Happy reader support group**.

Also, be sure to leave a review on the online store wherever you bought this cookbook and at Good Reads!

Whatever crisis you are going through, we are here to support you.

I can't wait to see you there!

Section 1
Meal Planning

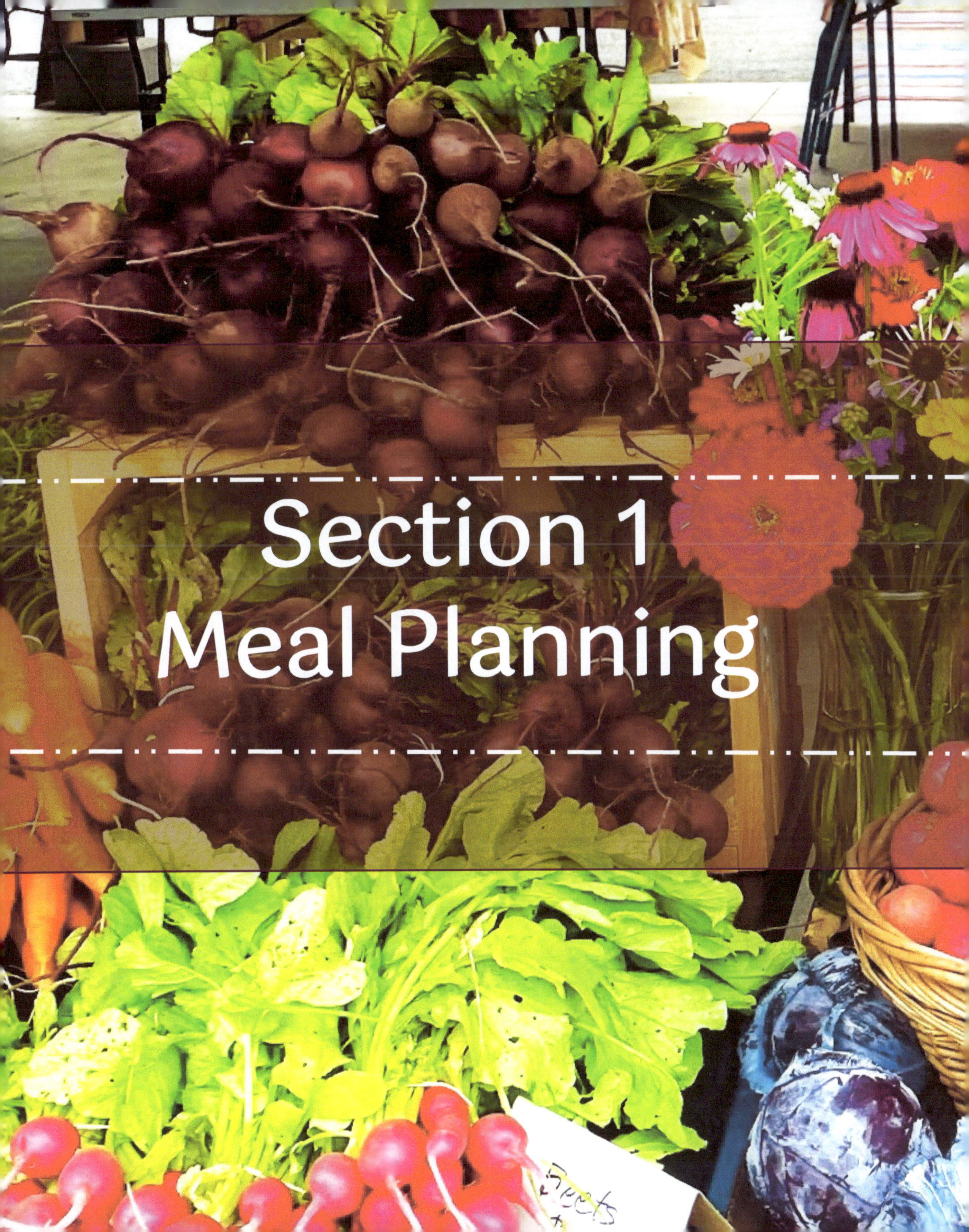

Menus

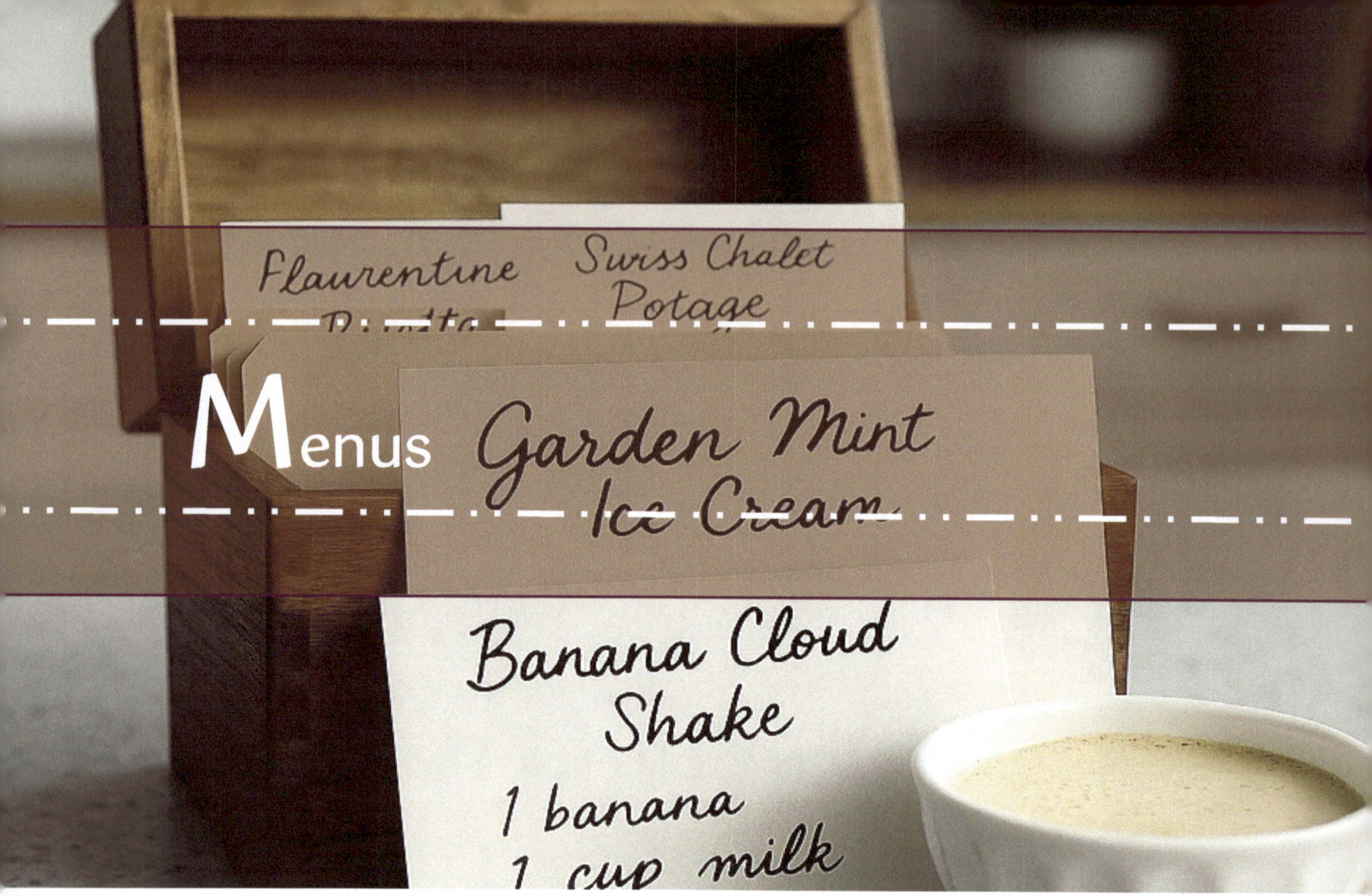

When you are having a hard day, you need to keep it simple. You need to be able to change plans in an instant. Even more importantly, you need to be forgiving of yourself.

Our bodies are designed not to eat very much when we are under a lot of stress or are very sick. Sometimes, our illnesses mean that we have symptoms flare when we eat.

We have to eat when we can. We have to eat what sounds appetizing.

We don't need to worry about whether it is breakfast time or dinner time. We don't need to be concerned about getting all of the food groups.

And we certainly don't need to be slaving over the stove for hours each day.

We need to do what we can do, and be grateful for that.

So, this cookbook is a little different. There are no menus. Although foods are divided into breakfasts, beverages, snacks, main courses, and desserts, take these divisions lightly. Cook and serve what you want to when you want to, and in whatever combinations you want to!

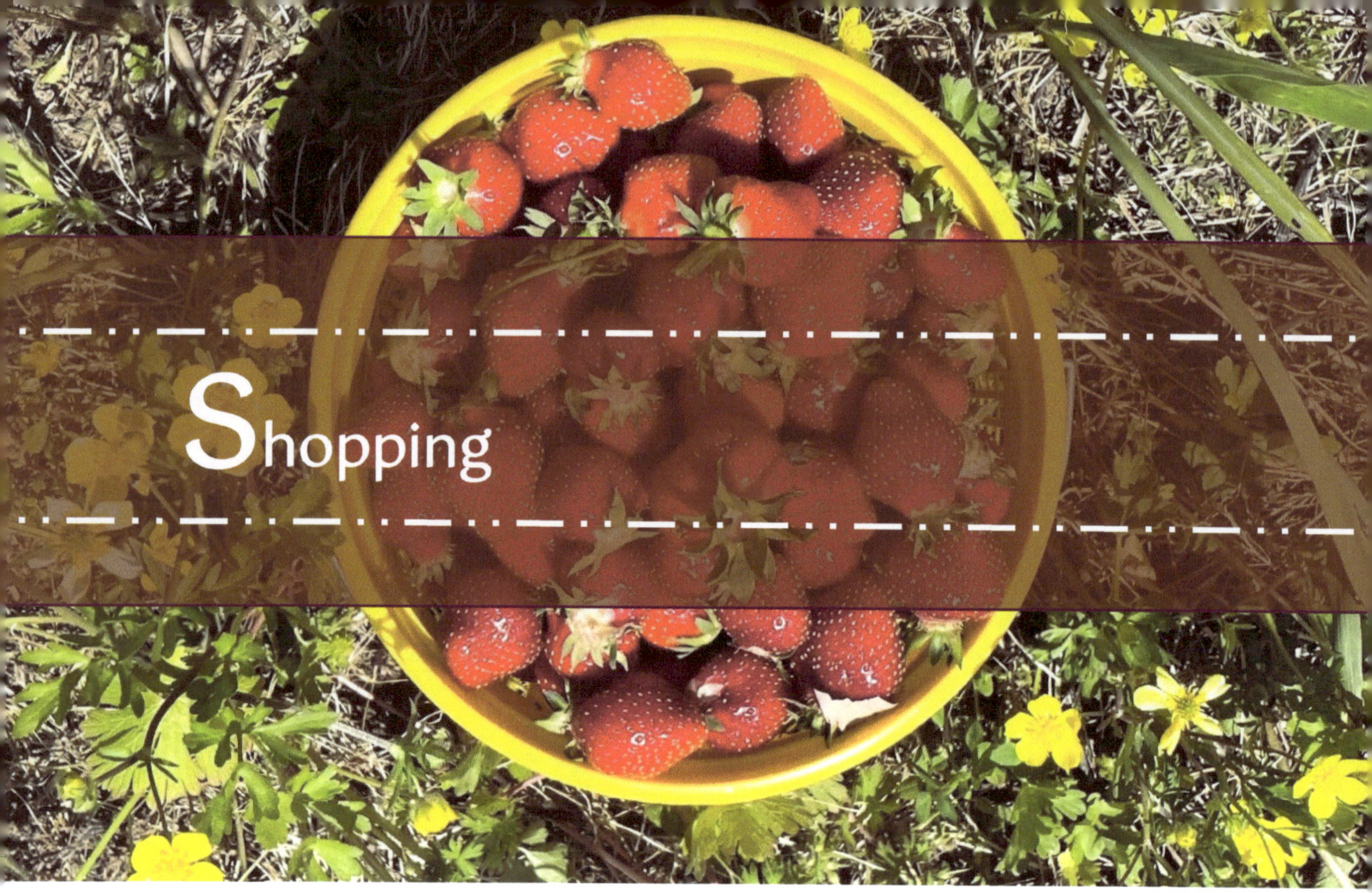

Shopping

Grocery Stores

If you are in a difficult season of life, grocery shopping is fraught with dangers and obstacles. Grocery stores are often very large, and the amount of walking required to traverse them is not feasible. Do not be afraid to use the provided electric scooter carts they keep plugged in at the front of the store.

Grocery stores are often kept very cold to keep the food fresh, so dress warmly and bring extra layers. If you start to get too cold, leave your half-full cart with the customer service desk and take a break outside. Sit in your car with the heater and seat warmers on if it's too cold outside. If you are going to need to take a break like this, try to get your freezer and refrigerator items at the end of your trip, regardless of where these aisles are in your store.

The smells in a grocery store are problematic for many people with chronic illnesses. Not only do grocery stores sell fragranced laundry products, candles, cleaning supplies, and toiletries, they use powerful cleaning products themselves. Wear a personal ionizer, and prepare your body for the potential exposure. My book *Hypermobile and Happy* contains a chapter on Allergies, MCAS, and MCS with many actionable suggestions for preparing for and coping with fragrance and chemical exposures.

Many people love going to the grocery store because they will get to bump into friends and acquaintances! This may be a benefit for you, as well, since you have been spending so much time at home alone, dealing with your personal crisis. However, it may be stressful for you if you are coping with symptoms and trying to make your trip as quick as possible. Find out when your grocery store offers specials for elderly customers, and try to go at that time. The store is usually less crowded, and everyone is a little more understanding and patient during these hours. When you do see someone you know, or when a stranger strikes up a conversation, simply answer politely: "It's nice to see you, but I am focused on my shopping because I need to make this trip as quick as possible."

Pick-Up and Delivery

When you are in crisis, delivery could be life-saving. Of course, there may be times when Door Dash or Uber Eats is your go-to delivery service, but your body will thank you when you discover grocery delivery and, even better, farmer delivery. The quality of foods from your grocery are superior to what most of the restaurants are offering, and your farmer's produce will be the freshest available.

Can you find someone locally who will bring a dozen eggs to your doorstep once a week? I guarantee they'll cost less than the organic eggs in the store, even though delivery is included. Pay with Venmo, and life is simple.

Many small farms are willing to deliver their products to your door whenever you place an order, or if you are a member of a CSA.

CSA (Community Supported Agriculture) shares are especially wonderful when you are healthy and cooking every day. With a CSA, generally you pay a farmer or group of farmers in advance of the harvest season, and then they provide you with a basketful of foods each week during the season. Where I live, CSAs of meat, dairy, and eggs are available year-round, and vegetable, fruit, and grain CSAs are offered all summer and fall.

CSAs always offer only the very best in freshness, quality, and variety. I especially appreciate that they inspire me to cook foods I otherwise wouldn't think to buy.

Another option is through your local farmer's market. Reach out to the organizer, and find out if you can order food in advance of the market and either do a curb-side pickup or get delivery. Many markets already have these options arranged, but if yours does not, the organizer may be willing to work with you and come up with ideas to help.

Among the many benefits of sourcing your food from local farms is the diminished risk of your food being treated with potentially harmful chemicals such as the invisible, tasteless coatings that are sprayed on most grocery-store produce to extend shelf life. Also, getting local food is the best way of getting fresh food, which also means that the produce does not have to withstand the rigors of extensive transportation, and so farmers are able to grow heritage varieties that are not selected for their shelf life and hardiness but rather for taste and high nutrient content.

U-Pick

If you have the time and ability to do some of the harvesting yourself, u-pick farms provide the ultimate in fresh food. This really matters if you have a histamine-sensitive condition like MCAS because histamine increases in produce as it ages. In addition to finding fresh produce at u-pick farms, you may find culinary weeds in your own yard or local wilderness park. Many of these foods are very high in nutrients.

Even better is growing a little bit of food yourself. This can be as simple as a small pot on your kitchen windowsill with an oregano or thyme plant that you can pull leaves off from time to time to drop into the food you're making.

Whether you are picking berries at a local farm or harvesting a tomato from your back porch, the time you spend in the fresh air and sunshine is going to be a bonus health boost. Most of the longest-lived people in the world get much of their exercise working in their garden.

Pantry Staples and Fresh Foods

Keep a list in your phone or your grocery store app of your staple foods. These should be the ingredients for your favorite recipes, snacks that require no cooking, and foods that are safe for you to eat even when you're at your worst. Make sure these are always on hand. It's a good idea to have 2 or 3 of each item so that there is 1 to eat and 1 to get you through until you make another shopping trip.

Staples should be foods that keep for a while, but the more health-giving foods will be the special ones that are in season. Even if you aren't able to get food directly from local farmers, the fresh produce in the grocery store that is on sale will likely be in season. As food is transported from the farms to the consumer, it ages, develops mold, increases in histamine content, and loses nutrient quality. Always aim to get the freshest, most local food you can find.

When fresh produce isn't available, organic frozen fruits and vegetables are the next best choice. In most cases, the food is frozen very soon after it is picked, so it will still be of high quality.

Quality Ingredients

At this time, organic is almost always a better choice than conventional.

Be aware that spices may develop mold inside the bottles. Also, spices are an ingredient that many people keep on their shelves long past their best-by dates. For these reasons, dried spices can be problematic for people with MCAS, other histamine issues, or mold illness.

I have had great success shopping for spices at Mountain Rose Herbs, even when I was very sensitive. An even better option is to keep a few pots of your favorite spice plants, like oregano, basil, and thyme, on your windowsill or porch. It can be difficult to keep plants alive when you are in crisis, but if watering them once a week can be part of your routine, you will be rewarded with really delicious, health-giving food, as these fresh spices are high in nutrients that are beneficial for healing symptoms like neuralgia, ligament injuries, and inflammation.

Food Prep

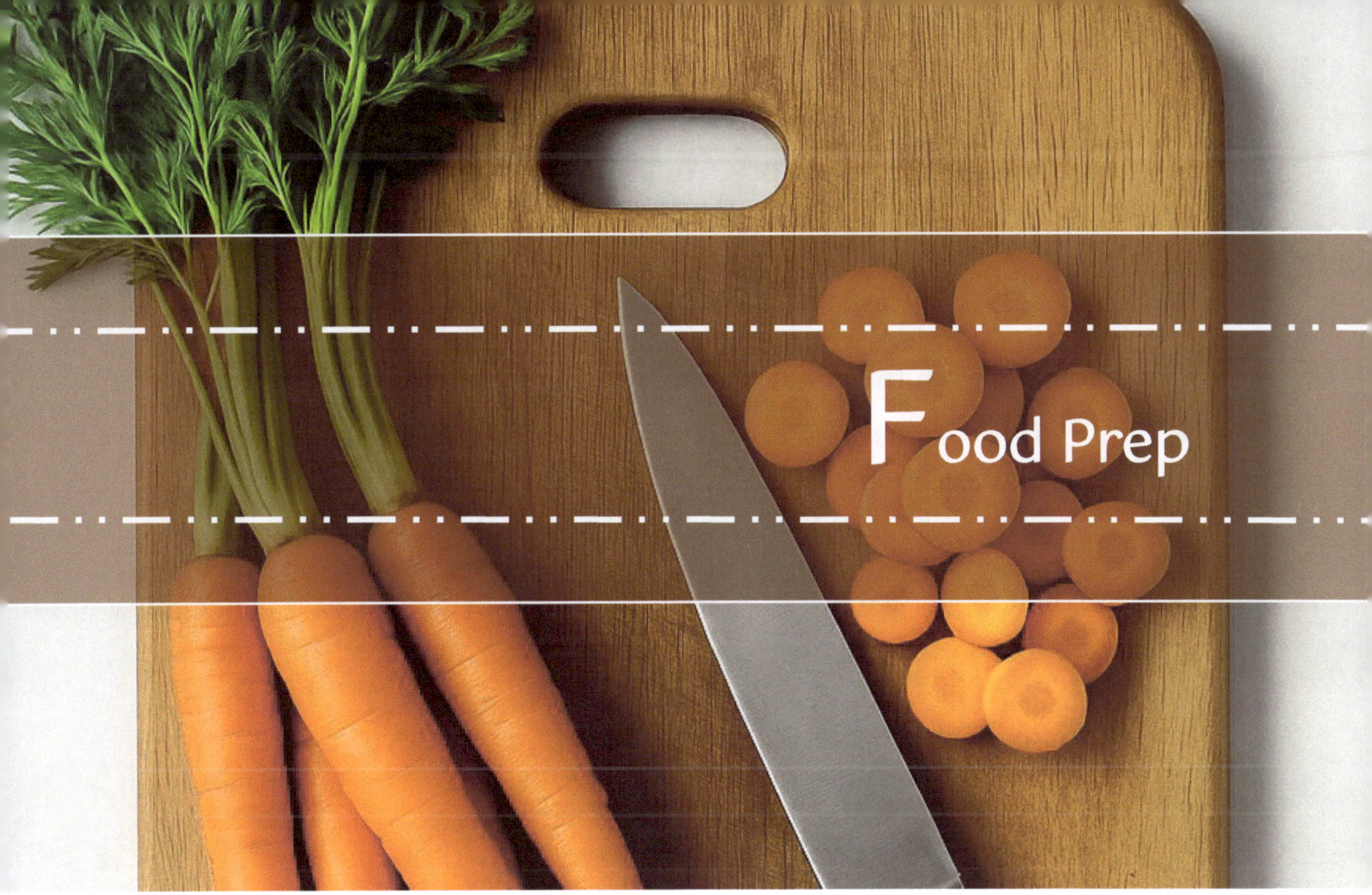

When you are under stress, coping with grief, or addled with worry, your mental efforts are using up all of your body's energy reserves. You just cannot devote hours to cooking each day. Even worse, depression and stress can cause physical symptoms to appear or become exacerbated in your body. If you already have a chronic condition, you can expect difficult situations to instigate symptom flares.

Chronic Illness Complicates Everything

Cooking on flare days is itself a recipe for a culinary disaster, and it can even be dangerous. Here are some of the most common symptoms I have experienced and heard my clients and readers complain about when it comes to cooking:

- Brain fog (poor memory, unclear thinking, difficulty making decisions, etc.) makes it hard to remember the steps of the processes you are doing.
- Mast Cell Activation Syndrome (MCAS) causes you to be sensitive to synthetic additives and pungent food ingredients. You also might get nauseated from the smell of foods that are cooking.
- Ataxia (incoordination caused by swelling in the brain) causes you to be too clumsy to safely do a lot of chopping or using the oven. You might spill things and break dishes frequently.
- Fibromyalgia (pain throughout the body) causes you to fatigue quickly when you work in the kitchen. Repetitive tasks are especially challenging.
- Postural Orthostatic Tachycardia Syndrome (POTS, characterized by racing heart, dizziness, nausea, trembling, weakness, etc.) causes you to have difficulty standing for a long period of time. You also might have wild body-temperature swings as you are intolerant of heat and cold, two conditions that exist in all kitchens.
- Attention Deficit Hyperactivity Disorder (ADHD) causes you to easily become over-stimulated by sensory inputs, bored by chores that you aren't passionate about, and easily distracted, sometimes forgetting about food that is cooking and ends up burnt.
- Ehlers-Danlos Syndrome or Hypermobility Spectrum Disorder (EDS or HSD, connective-tissue disorders characterized by overly flexible and unstable joints, causing symptoms in all of the systems of the body) causes you to easily injure your fingers, wrists, elbows, shoulders, neck, and any other joint in the body while cutting, carrying dishes, or doing repetitive tasks.

It is no surprise that people with chronic illnesses tend not to enjoy cooking, even though they need the homemade nourishment even more than most. Cuts, burns, bruises, aches, and fatigue are common after preparing a meal. Then, there's also the spills, broken dishes, and ruined foods you have to contend with. A bag of chips is sounding pretty good about now. But there is a better choice!

Use Supportive Tools

With this cookbook, you are going to find easy recipes that do not require a lot of chopping, standing at the kitchen counter for a long time, bending to pull items out of the oven, or manipulating skilled culinary techniques...but we can still make things even easier with supportive tools.

Many members of the chronic illness community on social media have reported that they love using a cushioned, rolling, saddle-seat stool in the kitchen. They are able to sit down while they cook, and their position allows them to move right up to the counter – and then roll around to the stove, sink, refrigerator, or pantry with ease.

A finger guard made of stainless steel is a tiny, inexpensive device that is imperative when chopping vegetables on a day when you're dealing with ataxia. There are other, larger but easier-to-use devices for cutting vegetables that I recommend if you have uncoordinated movements or joint injuries in the arms or hands on a regular basis. Buying pre-chopped fresh or frozen foods is the right option some of the time. Other times, using scissors instead of a knife is a safe choice.

Other must-have tools in the kitchen include a battery-operated pot stirrer, a jar opener, and an electric can opener.

You can find my product recommendations in my Amazon storefront in the Cooking Supplies list at https://bit.ly/4oNCVz3.

Advance Planning

Many people report that what works best for them is to chop all of their veggies as soon as they get them from the store. Some go even further, spending all day Sunday preparing all of the ingredients for each dish they are going to cook that week. If this works for you, you should definitely take advantage of that foresight and ability to get a lot done at once.

For many of us, though, a day of prep work is too exhausting...and too risky in the sense that we will likely not be able to stick to our meal plan for the full week. A flare day will happen, or maybe we simply won't have any appetite one day. It would be a shame for all of the ingredients and your time spent preparing them to go to waste because of this.

Additionally, anyone with histamine issues, such as those with MCAS, is potentially not going to do very well eating food that has been prepared and then sat in the fridge for days. As food ages, the histamine content increases; after it has been cut, mold can more readily take hold. This is not what we want, especially if we are going through a stressful time and our immune system is overactive.

Instead, use the recipes in this book for foods that do not take very much prep work in the first place. And, keep packages of pre-chopped frozen veggies in your freezer for use at a moment's notice.

Mise en place

Mise en place is a French term that translates, literally, as "put in place." It is the term chefs use to indicate that they have gathered all of their supplies and measured all of their ingredients before beginning to cook. Think about how TV chefs have everything they need in pretty little bowls at the beginning of each episode. They had a crew to do that work for them, though!

Working with *mise en place* is a good idea if you have a hard time walking or maneuvering on your rolling stool while you are cooking. Often, cooking requires precise timing and quick movements, so having everything together makes that easier.

What I find works better, though, is to rearrange your kitchen so that your *mise en place* is almost done for you before you even start. Store your spices, measuring spoons and cups, and cooking utensils close to the stove (but not so close that the heat of the stove will damage the spices). You don't have to keep food in your pantry and dishes in your cabinets – switch them around if that improves how easy it is to reach what you need while you're cooking.

One aspect of *mise en place* that I find to be particularly important, especially if brain fog, sadness, or distraction make it especially difficult for you to cook, is the policy of always reading the entire recipe before beginning to cook it.

You may need to read it a few times in order to notice everything and let it all sink in. You may need to read it again while in the midst of cooking. But the most important thing is just to read all the way through once before deciding to cook the recipe at all. (I'm looking at you, ADHD friends! I know you hate reading instructions, but you will be more successful if you do.)

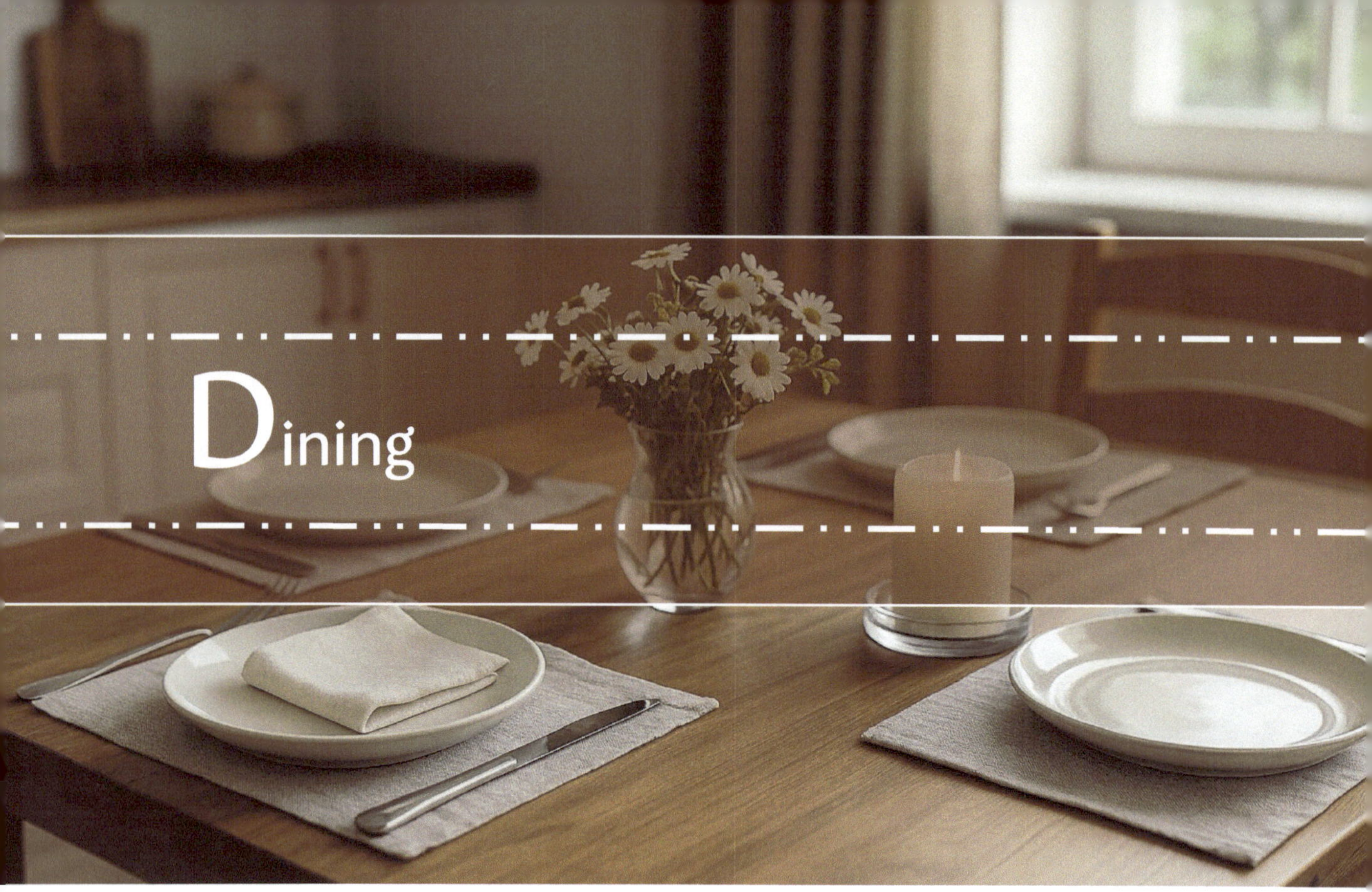

Dining

The recipes and ingredients are not the only things that matter when you eat. Timing, posture, and attitude can make a big difference in how health-giving your meal is.

Timing

When you are in crisis, eat when you can eat. Do not try to abide by traditional meal times. This isn't the time to give Intermittent Fasting or any other timing idea a try. Eat when you can, when you're hungry.

Whenever it is possible – you have a little extra energy or time – take steps to make your future meals and snacks more readily available. Ask friends to bring you single serving leftovers from their homes that you can put in the freezer. When a meal you cook has leftovers, put it in the freezer in single-serving sized microwave or oven-safe dish. Shop for snacks that can be kept in the freezer or on the shelf, ready whenever you are.

In addition to freezing leftovers, I like to freeze cupcakes and muffins. They defrost on the counter in about half an hour, and their taste and texture is just like fresh. One of the benefits of having cupcakes in the freezer is that if you are invited to a party where your food sensitivities will prevent you from partaking in what is served, you can take your own cupcake and be perfectly content.

For ready snacks, I keep frozen blueberries, which are delicious straight out of the freezer, and frozen edamame, which defrosts quickly on the counter and is quite tasty with salt, no cooking needed.

If you have help, you may benefit from using a stainless-steel, electric chafing dish. A loved one can put food into the dish in the morning, and it can stay fresh all day. Be aware, however, that if you have mast cell over-activation, the food may develop more histamine while in the dish, and your mast cells may get excited by the smell of the food in the air for a long period of time.

Nontoxic Dishes

Heat draws poisonous chemicals out of plastic dishes and deposits them into the foods that are touching the dishes, so it is best to usecom natural, inert choices like ceramic, stainless steel, and glass for cooking, serving, and dining. Even napkins should be made of soft cotton or a paper that feels good to the touch.

Disposable dishes can be an important time-and-effort saver for hard days, but make sure that they are paper (or sugar cane), not coated in plastic.

There are memes and community posts on social media regarding the perfect fork or spoon for people with autism, and there are some strong opinions about this. Even if you can get just one place setting for yourself, make sure that you enjoy the look and feel of each item you will touch during your meals. Beautiful dishes really can help us enjoy our food better. We sit up straighter, eat more slowly, and set ourselves up for good digestion, which is only going to benefit our healing journey.

If you are having trouble with cleanup after meals, eat over a table surface that you can easily wipe up with the napkin you were using. However, if you are experiencing sensory sensitivity, a placemat or tablecloth can dampen noises and feel comforting. A cushion on your dining chair and a footstool under the table can make you a lot more comfortable, too.

Posture

Digestion works best when gravity helps it along. Digestion also requires the imperceptible movement of internal organs – if they are too crowded due to poor posture, they may not be able to move the way they should. Of course, there are times when you may be ill and cannot sit up properly, but whenever possible, sit at a table, back straight, and looking at your food as you eat. Stay relaxed but activated.

There is a strong tradition in all societies for meals to be social occasions. This may benefit you if you are feeling lonely or weak. But if social interaction is too much for you, do not be afraid to eat alone. A book or television show makes a fine companion, too, though it is best if you put your attention on the food. However, pay attention to your posture when eating alone.

Our posture changes when we are around different people – sometimes for the better and sometimes for the worse. It is hard to pay attention to posture at the same time as paying attention to your friend and eating. Don't worry about it. But when you eat alone, you can spare some attention for your posture, which is good since a lot of people (especially you hypermobile ones) relax, let go...and start slouching when they are alone. If your shoulders roll forward and your back curves while you're eating, there will not be room for your esophagus, stomach, and intestines to do the work they are supposed to do. It is very important for your digestive health that you sit up straight while you eat. Even standing is better than slouching on the sofa.

Attitude

The most overlooked and yet potentially most important aspect of nutrition is your attitude toward it. Scientists have found that food has different actions and measurable health outcomes in the body depending on your frame of mind when you are eating it.

If you know that your food is full of nutrition and health-giving constituents, your food will do your body good. If you know that what you're eating is saturated in poisonous chemicals and void of vitamins and minerals, your health may suffer for it. So, first of all, choose healthy foods, and secondly, tell yourself that this food will bring you health.

Prepare your food with gratitude for it. Pay attention to the color, smell, texture, and magnificent miracle it is that it could grow, be harvested, and find its way to your kitchen. Hold yourself in reverence for the earth, sun, rain, wind, birdsong, farmer, pollinating insects, truck driver, grocer, and your own luck of being able to afford and prepare this food. It is quite a blessing that so much has happened right so that you have the pleasure of a meal.

Have you ever thought about the hands that have touched your food before it got to you? It is somewhat common for prayers before meals to acknowledge the hands that prepared the food...but this does not only include the person in the kitchen. Your food was also touched by a farmer and possibly a trucker, a grocer, and numerous others.

It is a very good idea to express your gratitude and intention for the meal aloud. If you have a spiritual or religious tradition of prayer, invoke it wholeheartedly, and imagine the sense of nourishment, fortification, and wellbeing this meal will provide. There are many traditional grace prayers to be found online, or make up your own. I will put a few at the end of the next section, under Spiritual Nourishment.

Cleaning Up

It is important not to let dirty dishes and uneaten food clutter your home. The smells and appearance will not improve your appetite.

My number one recommendation when you are in crisis is to use disposable tableware as much as possible, and throw it away when you are done eating. This is not the time to be environmentally conscientious. However, it would be wise to use uncoated paper dishes so that your food does not absorb the plastics of the coatings of typical disposable tableware. Paper and sugarcane options can easily be found online even if they are not in your local grocery store.

Most of the time for most people, I do not recommend putting very many leftovers in the refrigerator, if any at all. During a crisis, your meal opportunities and appetite are too unreliable; the refrigerated food is likely to go bad and just become another chore to deal with. Mold grows even in the refrigerator and can cause allergic-like symptoms. Freezing leftovers in single-serving dishes works better for many foods.

Do not be afraid to ask a loved one to help with the cleaning up. If you can afford to hire someone to come in and clean house on a regular basis, this will help you maintain a positive mood throughout the crisis period.

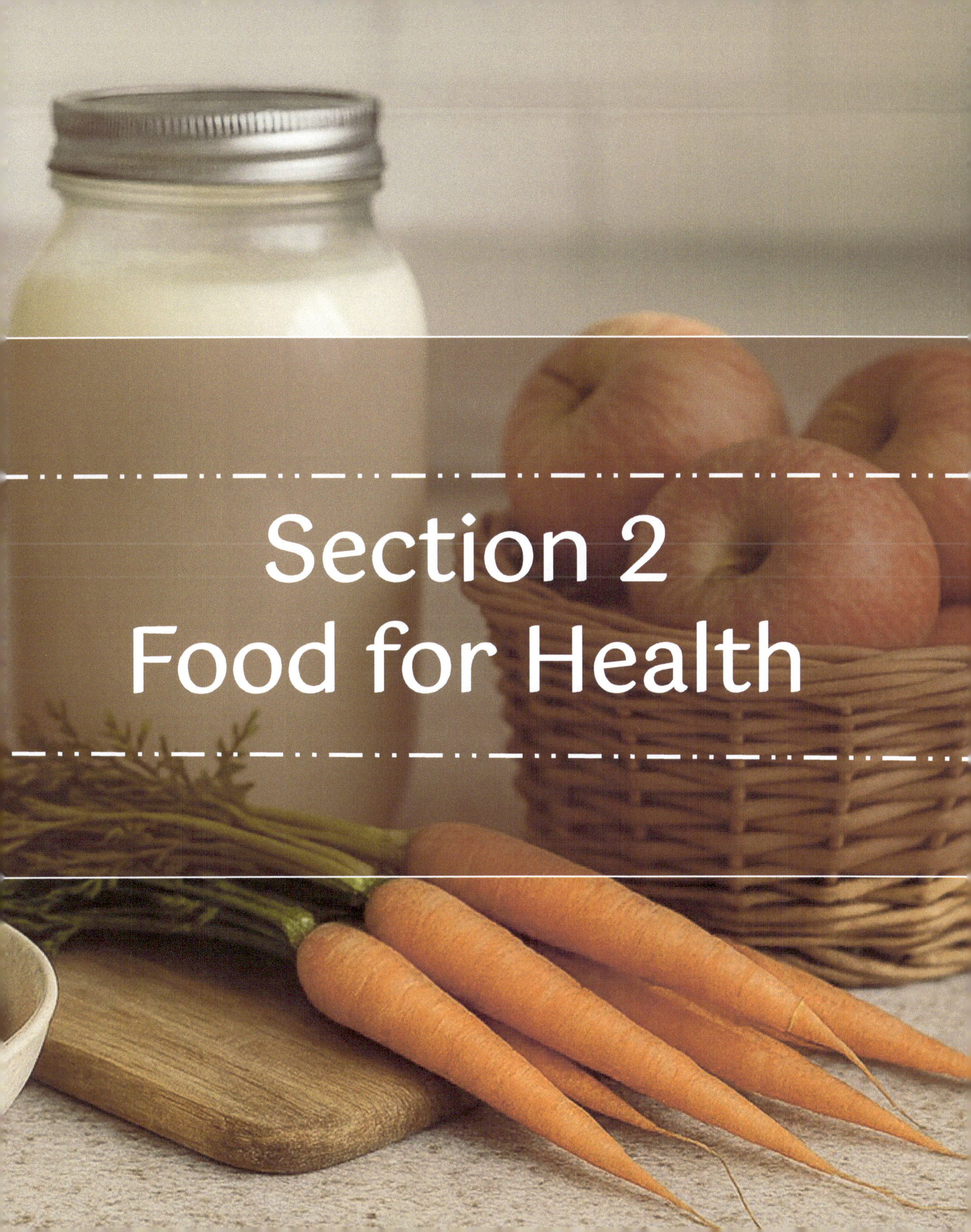

Section 2
Food for Health

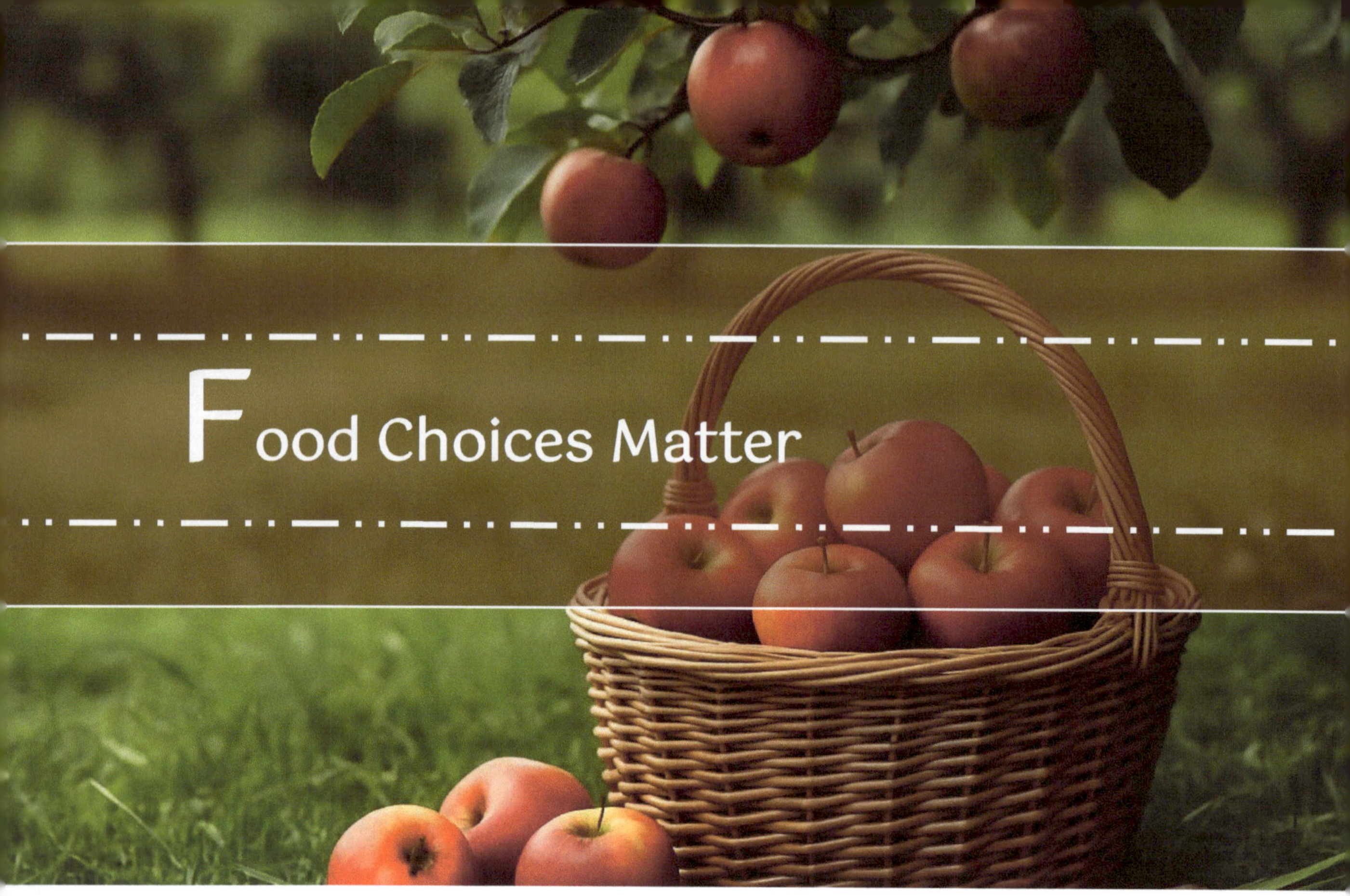

Food Choices Matter

Food choices matter when you're in crisis. The stress on your body during a crisis, even if it's a mental, psychological, or emotional crisis, can make your body more susceptible to developing diseases, experiencing symptom flares, or reacting poorly to foods. For this reason, it is important to choose health-giving ingredients.

Ingredients to Watch Out For

Did you know that food dyes, artificial flavors, preservatives, and most synthetic food additives are made from petroleum? This is a poison, so it is no wonder that it creates havoc on our health over the long term.

Most produce that is conventionally grown is treated with pesticides and other chemicals that are poisonous to humans. It is best to choose organic whenever you possibly can.

There are also components that naturally occur in foods that are problematic for some people, especially during times of crisis. I recommend that you search online for the symptoms and food lists for foods that contain:

- high histamine
- gluten
- alkaloids (nightshades)
- oxalates
- salicylates
- tannins
- common allergens
- aged foods (dried, fermented, or preserved)

If you react badly to any of these families of foods, you will want to avoid them until you are in better health.

A food diary can be very helpful in determining which foods are good or bad for your body at this time. Keep in mind that it can change over time! I have created the *Hypermobile and Happy Health Diary* as an easy tool for keeping comprehensive records of your symptoms and food intake. You can purchase it at www.shannonegale.com. Fill it out for 6 weeks and see if any patterns become apparent.

A Well-Rounded Diet is Important

Many people with unrecognized and untreated MCAS are limited to a very small number of foods. Even if they are eating a normal serving size at every meal, they lose weight and watch their health deteriorate because they are missing vital nutrients.

Another benefit of a well-rounded diet is how food combinations work. This is very complex, but fortunately, we traditionally eat foods in combinations that are optimized for nutrition; they taste better in those combinations, too.

For example, when you put butter on your baked potato, the fat will assist the body in absorbing the vitamins in the potato. Beans and rice together make a complete protein. When you enjoy cheddar cheese with apple slices, the high fiber content of the apple will bind the histamine of the cheese and reduce the body's absorption of the histamine.

Easy to Digest Meals

During chronic illness and times of stress, the digestive system may not be working optimally. We will do best if we offer our bodies food that is easy to digest. There are two main ways in which the recipes in this cookbook accomplish that:

1. Food that is cooked thoroughly and is warm, and
2. Food that is liquid.

Ingredients that are cooked have already had their proteins begin to unravel and cell walls begin to break down so that the core nutrients are easier to extract. Also, the digestive system requires heat to do its work, so warm foods make it easier.

Foods that are liquid (beverages and soups) are also easy to digest, as if they have already been thoroughly chewed and partially broken down by stomach acids. This is especially important for anyone with gastroparesis, a condition more common among those with hypermobility in which stomach emptying is uncomfortably and problematically delayed. Liquids have a much faster rate of gastric emptying than solids do.

No matter what you are eating, you can also help the digestive process by chewing your food thoroughly. When in a season of stress, you are likely to gulp down food quickly, which only leads to stomach aches and decreased nutrient absorption. Slow down, and chew your food until it is fluid.

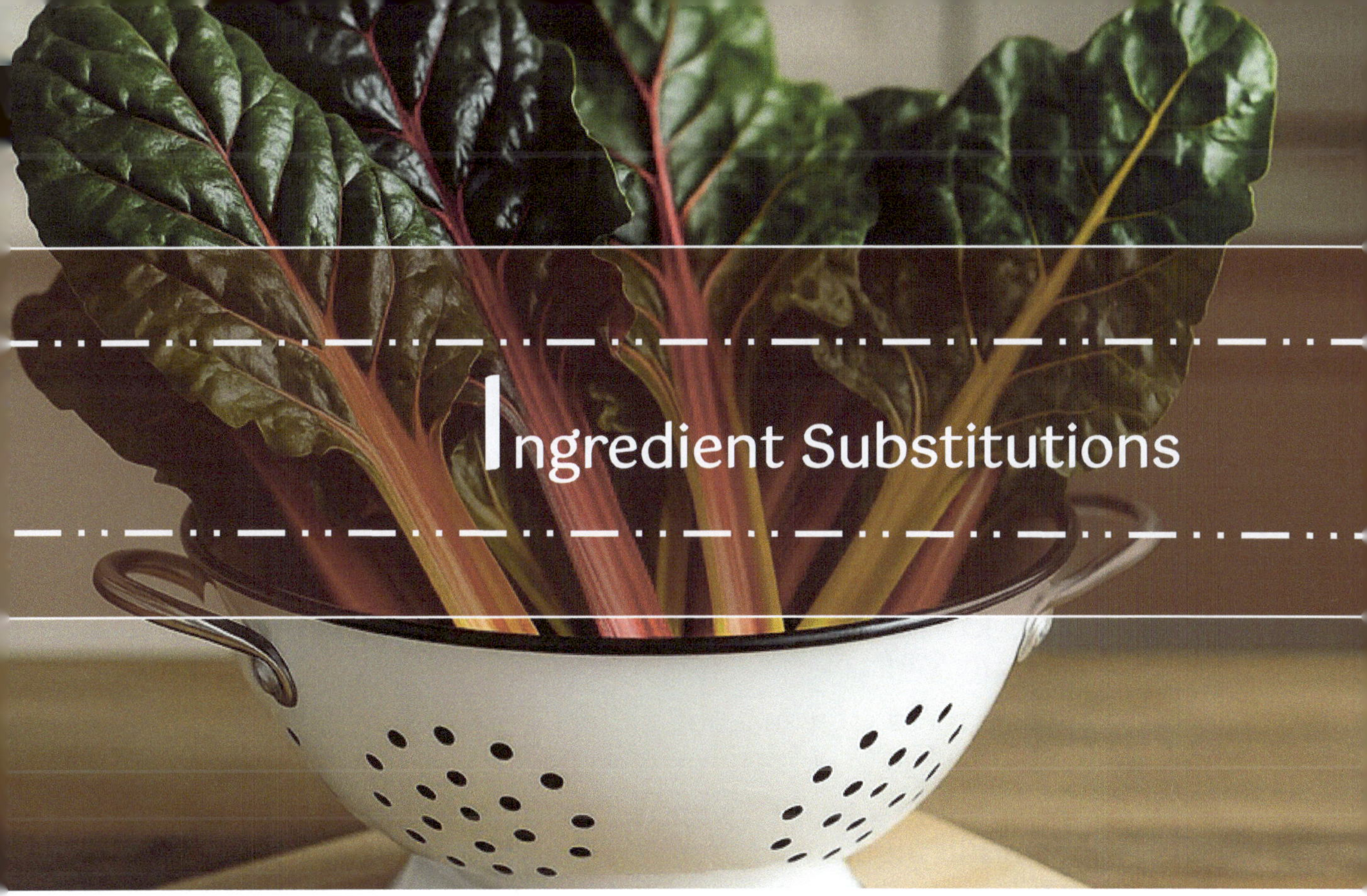

Ingredient Substitutions

There are some ingredients listed in this cookbook in simplistic form because any version of them will do, but I'd like to explain how to get the best flavors and health-giving properties by making specific choices.

Immune Boosting Foods

Many people with chronic illness, autoimmune diseases, allergies, and stress have heightened immune systems. During this time, it is best to avoid foods that rally the immune system. Garlic, onions, and spicy peppers are among these foods. At other times, when you are trying to fight off a cold or flu, eat extras of these foods, especially in their raw state. Cooking will diminish (or change) their immune-boosting properties a little bit.

For the most part, I have left these commonly used immune-boosting foods out of the recipes, even though a huge percentage of today's popular recipes are based on garlic, onions, and hot or bell peppers. This cookbook is special in highlighting other flavors for more diversity in your repertoire.

Sometimes the flavors of these ingredients are still desirable, and so you will find them in some of the recipes in this book. Use them only when you feel that your immune system is calm enough to handle them. When you do eat them, pay attention so that you can notice if you become more reactive and sensitive.

In order to get the same flavor with somewhat less potency, you can substitute leeks or chives for onions, bell peppers for spicy peppers, and garlic scapes for garlic cloves.

Chives are easy to grow in a pot and need little, if any care. You can simply snip off a leaf or several leaves as needed; the plant will be fine.

If you remove the seeds and white spines of bell peppers, they will be less problematic. Also, avoid green peppers, as they are actually just unripe red (or orange, yellow, or purple) peppers. Paprika is dried and ground red bell peppers, and sometimes it is a nice substitution.

Garlic scapes are a green part of the garlic plant – the stem that grows tall in the spring and, if not picked to be eaten, develops a flower bloom at the top. Many farmers harvest garlic scapes because the bulbs will grow better if the plant is not allowed to flower. The scapes are much milder than the cloves, but their flavor and texture are delightful.

Milk

I always use raw whole milk that I get directly from a farmer. It has been thought that milk needs to be pasteurized to be safe to drink, but that is because milk from cows on conventional farms is not safe. On those farms, cows are raised in filthy, inhumane conditions without sufficient (or any) access to pasture to get the nutrients, exercise, and sunlight they need.

Raw milk dairies are very different. I have visited my dairy farmer's land and seen how happy his cows are in their beautiful, large pastures. They even have a donkey with an amusing personality to keep them company. Birds, rabbits, butterflies, and other wildlife are their friends. But their favorite friend is the gentle farmer. Every morning, they amble to the barn to meet him there, knowing that he will give them a little bit of organic grain while he milks them. He is also very cautious about following the very best practices for keeping the milk safe from contamination.

Raw milk is not only safe, it is very good for you. It contains beneficial enzymes, diverse probiotics, healthy fats and proteins, bioavailable vitamins and minerals, immunoglobins, and other important nutrients. It also tastes delicious.

There is no way you will get the rich, wonderful flavor of raw milk from any other kind of milk. However, if you do not live near a small, organic dairy farm, an organic whole milk from the grocery store is your best bet.

If for any reason you wish to avoid dairy products, any other kind of "milk" will do. I have, from time to time, made the recipes in this book using soy milk, almond milk, oat milk, and cashew milk, though I caution you to be aware of added ingredients in most brands of these milks.

Gluten

Many people with EDS and autoimmune diseases are sensitive to, allergic to, or intolerant of gluten, the main protein found in wheat products. This may be because conventionally grown wheat is sprayed with glyphosate products shortly before harvesting because it dries out the wheat so that it can better be harvested. This poison is not washed off of the wheat, not even by rain, so conventional wheat products are very high in poison.

Additionally, until the modern era, humans almost always ate wheat after it had been fermented, such as for sourdough bread. The fermentation process partially breaks down the gluten. For this reason, some people who cannot tolerate typical wheat products are able to eat organic sourdough bread, especially if it is made with freshly milled wheat. Flour begins to go bad almost as soon as it has been milled, which is especially a problem for people with MCAS.

For the recipes in this cookbook, all of the breads or pastas can easily be replaced with whatever gluten-free options you prefer.

Not-Lean Meat

For many years, people have been avoiding fat and choosing lean meat in an attempt to be healthier, but the science has been showing that fat is important. Our brains are made of 60% fat. Traditionally, the Native American people valued fat in their diets above all other nutrients.

Fat is high in calories, which can be detrimental to a weight loss program, but even when losing weight, fat is a necessary part of the diet. As long as you are not overindulging in sugary sodas or processed foods replete with seed oils, it will be very unlikely that you will desire to eat more fat than is good for you. Even saturated fat from animals, long vilified, is now being found to be a beneficial part of the diet.

Fatty meats will make your meals taste better and be more satisfying. I almost always choose chicken thighs rather than breasts and local organic beef that is not exclusively grass fed, as small amounts of organic grains in the animals' diets leads to a better ratio of fat and better flavor in the meat.

Meats can be a very important part of a healthy diet. They contain complete proteins – no careful food combining necessary. They also have bioavailable vitamins and minerals, including some that cannot be found in vegetables, like B12. Early humans likely got much of their B12 from water, but now that we drink treated water, that is not an option for us.

Meat also has other compounds that cannot be found in plant foods, such as creatine, taurine, carnosine, and D3. Beef can be especially helpful for people with hypermobility and POTS due to its high protein content, as well as heme iron and B vitamins that help maintain blood volume and heal nerve damage.

When choosing meats to eat, it is extremely important to pick organic meat, preferably from a small, local farm. Conventional meat farming practices are abhorrent. If the only meat you can get is conventional, you may be better off abstaining from eating it.

I like to visit the farms where I get my meat and see that the animals are raised in the open air in a natural setting. I always find that the farmers are kind and respectful of the animals as well.

Although meat is generally a healthy choice, if you prefer not to eat it ever or on a certain day, it can easily be left out of the recipes in this cookbook. Aside from Tender Pot Chicken, my family has, at times, enjoyed each of the recipes in vegetarian form. Even the Easy Pot Roast Stew sometime gets re-imagined and renamed Pot Roastless Vegetables.

Fats

Fats, and especially saturated fats, have been given a bad rap for the past few decades, but recent research has been finding that they are incredibly important for our health.

Fats form the structural foundation of every cell membrane. The myelin sheath of nerves, which is essential for the nerves to be able to send their electric signals, is rich in fats, especially cholesterol, so saturated fats are essential for the proper operation of the nervous system.

Fats are required for the body to absorb certain vitamins and synthesize hormones. Without enough fat, we experience mood swings, blood-sugar instability, and physiological stress. The mitochondria, which are the energy-producing generators of the body's cells, require fat in order to power muscles, the brain, and the autonomic system.

People with hypermobility are prone to compression syndromes in which the skeletal and fascial systems do not hold the body in optimal postures, allowing blood vessels and nerves to be compressed. This is exacerbated in people who are too lean because they do not have fat cushioning the blood vessels and nerves.

Butter is a fat that may be especially important for people with hypermobility because of its important role in keeping the gut barrier from being "leaky." One of the components of butter, butyric acid or butyrate, is a fatty acid that is named for butter and is one of the most important chemicals for intestinal health. The bacteria in your gut can create butyrate when they break down fruits, vegetables, grains, and legumes. Your body can also use the butyrate from dairy products.

In recent decades, seed oils have been hyped to the exclusion of saturated fats (which come from animals), but our population's poor health is a testament to the error of this stance. In particular, seed oils turn out to contribute to chronic inflammation and cause damage to our cells. Seed oils are created through industrial processes that require the use of toxic chemicals and result in oils that are unstable and quickly go rancid.

An oil that deserves attention because it is a plant oil but not a seed oil is avocado oil. Whereas olive oil has been produced and eaten for millennia, avocado oil is new; because of this, regulations are, as of yet, not as strict as for olive oil. Although avocado oil may be a healthy and tasty choice, it might be made with rotting avocados that were not fit to be sold as produce in grocery stores, adulterated with other types of oil (some bottles labeled avocado oil have been found to be entirely soybean oil), or rancid before its expiration date due to improper processing methods. On the other hand, olive growers choose species specifically for oil production; although they sell some olives for eating, they are not making their oil out of fruits that would otherwise be thrown away. Not too long ago, olive oil labeling was not strictly standardized, but it is much more reliable now and generally a healthy choice.

Each cooking fat has different benefits and limitations; for example, butter is delicious but burns at lower temperatures than other animal fats. Tallow and bacon grease are good for high-heat cooking but can impart meat flavors to foods, though tallow's flavor is very subtle and often unnoticeable. Olive oil should not be heated beyond low heat and is best added to the serving plate after cooking has finished, but it can add a delicious flavor and feel to many dishes.

For some people, especially during chronic illness, fats can be difficult to digest. When this is the case, it is possible to sauté foods in a small amount of water.

My family almost always chooses butter, tallow, bacon grease, and olive oil to serve as the fats in our cooking processes. Lard and coconut oil are also good choices, though coconut oil goes through an intense refining process that makes it a suboptimal choice for some people.

The recipes in this book often do not specify the type of fat to be used so that you can choose what is easiest and tastiest for you. My family always has bacon grease that has been drained from breakfast preparations, filtered through a stainless-steel sieve, and stored in the refrigerator, so it serves as the basis for much of my cooking. You can always substitute the fats in these recipes in whatever way suits you best.

Broth

Many of the recipes in this cookbook call for broth. You can use homemade or storebought broths or stocks, or you can use bouillon cubes or pastes – whatever you prefer!

Homemade bone broth made with organic bones is extraordinarily health giving and full of the amino acids, collagen peptides, and electrolytes that everyone, but especially anyone with EDS, really needs. However, some people with MCAS are bothered by foods that are cooked over such long periods of time. I find that a homemade organic bone broth that is made with some of the fat from the meat in the pot is the best choice for me. When it cools, the fat forms a seal on top of the broth, which preserves it so that I will not have an MCAS reaction to it. However, I also opt for store-bought broth in glass jars when I don't have an opportunity to make homemade.

Real Maple Syrup

In place of white sugar, I almost always choose real maple syrup, which is made by boiling the sap of the maple tree. Honey, agave syrup, coconut sugar, regular sugar, turbinado sugar, date sugar, xylitol, stevia, or any sweetener of your choice could serve as substitutes for maple syrup, though the liquid content of the recipe may need to be adjusted by adding a little water. Most of the time, a 1 to 1 substitution will work out fine.

Maple syrup has a delicious flavor, is easy to use, has a low glycemic load, contains important vitamins and minerals, and is the only source in the world of certain beneficial compounds that are especially helpful for modulating and strengthening the immune system.

I purchase maple syrup at a local farm where I have been able to witness the entire process of tapping the trees, harvesting sap, cooking the sap over a wood fire, filtering it using an antique machine, and bottling the resulting thick, dark syrup by hand. This substance is very different from the pancake syrup available in grocery stores, which is made mostly of corn syrup.

If maple syrup does not work for you for any reason, it is easily substituted 1 to 1 with honey. Try to find a local, organic, raw honey. Note that most states do not have laws about what constitutes "local," so you may want to talk to your beekeeper to find out where their honey comes from.

Berries

You will notice that I include berries in several recipes. They are delicious, easy to use, and very good for us. As their bright colors communicate to us, they are full of antioxidants, which protect our cells from damage.

If you have MCAS, you need to be careful because berries mold more quickly than other fruits. I prefer to pick them myself at U-Pick farms or local wilderness parks because then I have the freshest berries possible. Frozen berries from the grocery store are also a good choice.

In addition to having high antioxidant content, blueberries help balance blood sugars, which can reduce symptoms in POTS patients. Their action is so strong that people with Type I diabetes who begin eating blueberries every day are able to reduce the amount of insulin they must take.

All of the berry recipes in this book indicate a specific berry that I prefer for this use. However, they are all interchangeable, and other berries, like blackberries, mulberries, cherries, and huckleberries would work just as well.

Spices

In this cookbook, I have not gone overboard recommending spices because many people with MCAS react to them due to high histamine or mold content. However, fresh herbs are almost always good for us. In fact, in *Hypermobile and Happy*, some of the recommended healing treatments were specific plants that are used to spice our food. All fresh spices are good for you, and dried spices that are stored correctly are, too (especially if you do not have MCAS), so season your food liberally.

I have recommended my favorite spices for the recipes in this book, but feel free to substitute your own instead. Changing spices will change flavor but not the consistency or cooking qualities of any of these dishes. Keep your favorite seasoning herbs growing in pots in your kitchen windowsill, and you'll be able to put a few fresh leaves into whatever you are cooking.

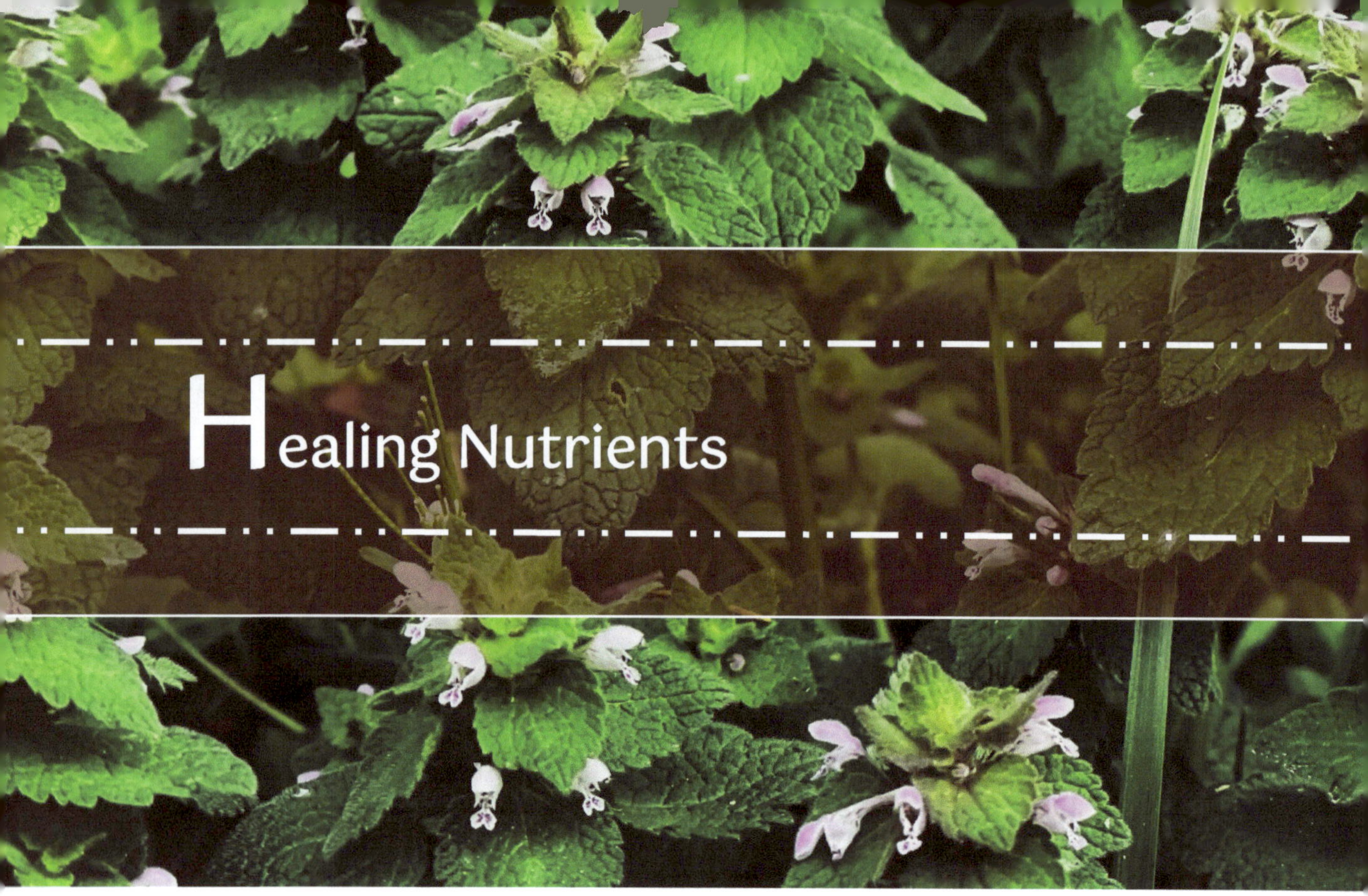

Healing Nutrients

Food can be one of your most important healing agents. Many of the medicines on the market today are simply mimicking, sometimes multiplying, the healing powers of foods.

If you are eating a real-food diet made at home with whole-food ingredients, it is likely that every single bite you take is healing. All plant and animal foods contain elements that our bodies need, and as long as you are not confusing your body with processed foods, you probably crave the nutrition your body needs. This makes eating healthy very easy.

If you are going through stress or have a chronic illness, there are certain foods you should try and see if they make a difference to you. If you haven't tried them recently, your body may not know to crave the taste of them. Eat them a few times and see if you desire to make them part of your regular meal rotation.

Most foods are really good for us. If you are choosing organic, unprocessed ingredients, you can assume that every food you choose is going to be good for you.

Based on the research I have done regarding agricultural processes, I choose to eat organic, local, raw milk, butter, and cheese; homemade bone broth; true sourdough bread made with freshly-milled wheat flour; other organic grains; local eggs raised by a friend whose chickens have the run of her large yard; organic, local, pasture-raised meats and animal fats; biodynamic-grown local vegetables and fruits; foraged fruits, vegetables, and herbs; and wild seafood and game.

Depending on your needs, you can focus your menu choices at any time. Look online for lists of foods that are:

- Anti-inflammatory
- Mast-cell stabilizers
- Prebiotics and probiotics
- Rich in specific vitamins and minerals

If you haven't read the previous section, Ingredient Substitutions, go back to it and pay attention to the beneficial qualities that are mentioned for each of the ingredients. They might serve some of your health needs.

I especially urge you to read my book, *Hypermobile and Happy*. It gives specific recommendations for foods and herbs that are scientifically proven to be effective at healing certain symptoms and conditions. It also includes exercises, lifestyle changes, alternative healing techniques, and more to support your health in a natural, holistic way.

Chocolate

One of the healing nutrients that I want to give special attention to is chocolate. We think of chocolate as an indulgent treat, but in fact, the fruit of the cacao plant, from which cocoa powder is made and then turned into chocolate, is very good for us.

Scientists have found that cocoa significantly improves blood flow, especially to the extremities. It also reduces inflammation because it is rich in flavanols. These compounds additionally increase nitric oxide levels in the blood, which improves blood flow, relieves brain fog, quickens recovery from exercise, reduces cold hands and feet, and can even improve vascular tone, possibly alleviating POTS symptoms.

Chocolate has compounds that stimulate the body's production of serotonin, dopamine, endorphins, and other chemicals, improving mood and reducing feelings of stress and anxiety. Cocoa is also one of the highest natural sources of magnesium, a mineral that many people with chronic illness are deficient in. Magnesium relaxes muscles, maintains nerve function, improves sleep quality, and relieves headaches, cramping, and other types of pain. The body uses extra magnesium during times of stress, so be sure you are getting enough when you are in crisis.

Cacao is extremely high in antioxidants, which protect collagen, joints, blood vessels, the nervous system, and more. Cocoa also contains polyphenols, which act as prebiotics to feed beneficial gut bacteria.

Unfortunately, most of the chocolate candies and hot cocoa mixes for sale in the grocery stores contain unhealthy ingredients, such as seed oils, corn syrup, ultra-processed sugars, artificial flavors (which are made from petroleum), emulsifiers like soy lecithin (that are bad for gut health), preservatives like TBHQ (that are linked to inflammation), hydrogenated oils (that are bad for cardiovascular health), and anti-caking agents like carrageenan and diglycerides.

Pure, organic chocolate products in the grocery store are usually pretty expensive. You can make even tastier options at home with easy-to-find organic cocoa powder. You'll be surprised how simple and rewarding this is!

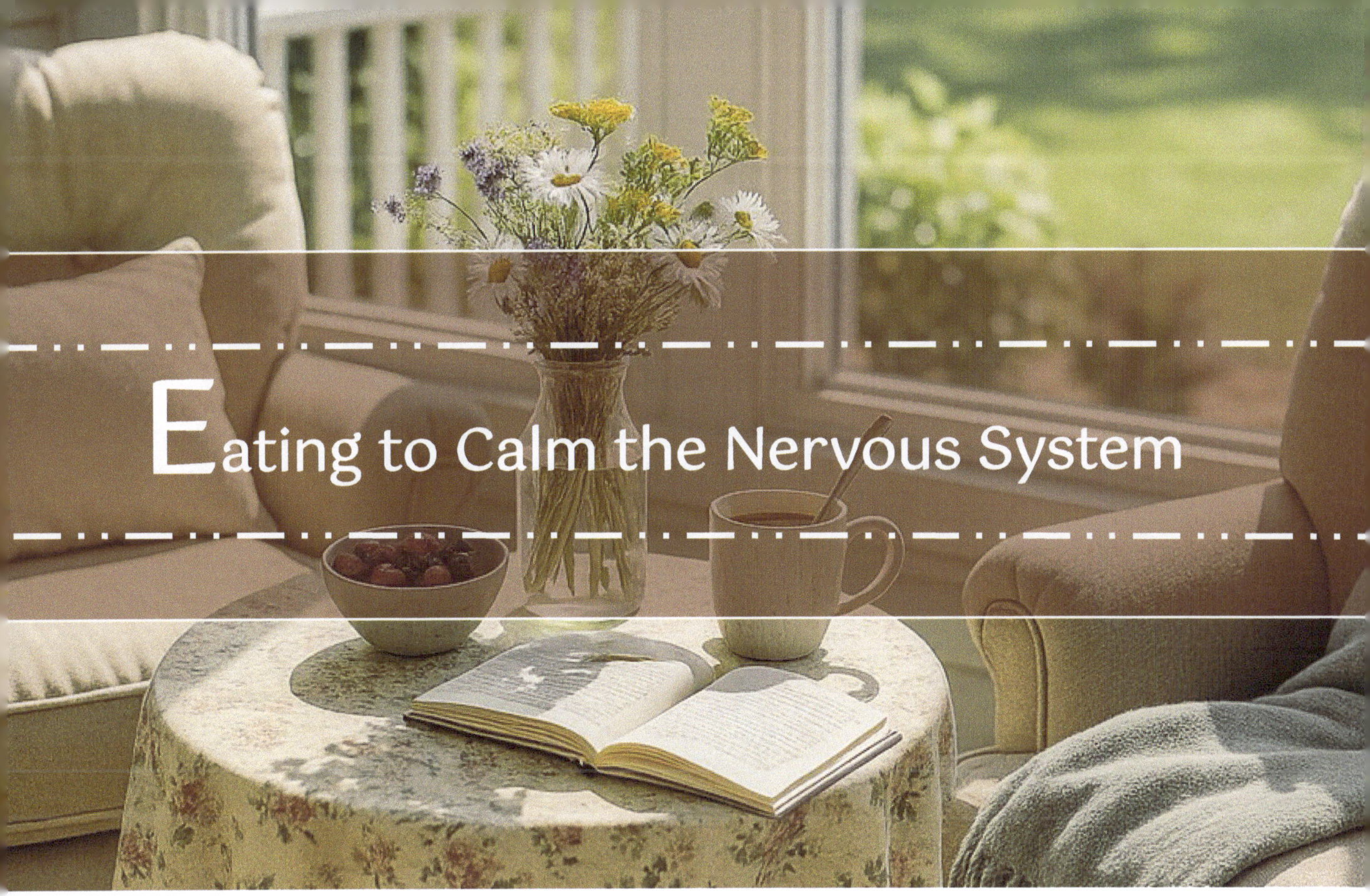

Eating to Calm the Nervous System

If you are in a moment of crisis, your Sympathetic Nervous System (SNS) is probably activated. The SNS is part of the autonomic nervous system, and it activates when a fight-or-flight response is needed to protect you from a threat. When in this state, the Parasympathetic Nervous System cannot fulfill the functions of digesting, healing, and recovering.

In addition to the SNS calling the shots, when you are in crisis, your nervous system becomes overactive. It will be hypervigilant, on high alert to make sure that it notices and reacts to any danger – large, small, or only perceived.

Interestingly, eating is one of the ways you can calm your nervous system down and get back into the rest and digest state. Unfortunately, it is not always sufficient for this purpose. There are many other natural and holistic techniques to do this, some of which are discussed in the chapter on Vagus Nerve Stimulation in *Hypermobile and Happy*. We will focus on eating here.

Eating should be a very enjoyable way of affecting your nervous system. Enjoying anything is beneficial for your nervous system, and if you're taking time to have a meal, that is a clear message to your body that you are safe, for the moment at least.

The act of chewing and sucking is also beneficial for the nervous system. The rhythmic movements of the mouth increase blood flow to the brain. Certain areas of the brain are stimulated, while others are calmed. Chewing can decrease levels of cortisol (a stress hormone) and help the body switch out of the Sympathetic Nervous System activation and into the rest-and-digest state.

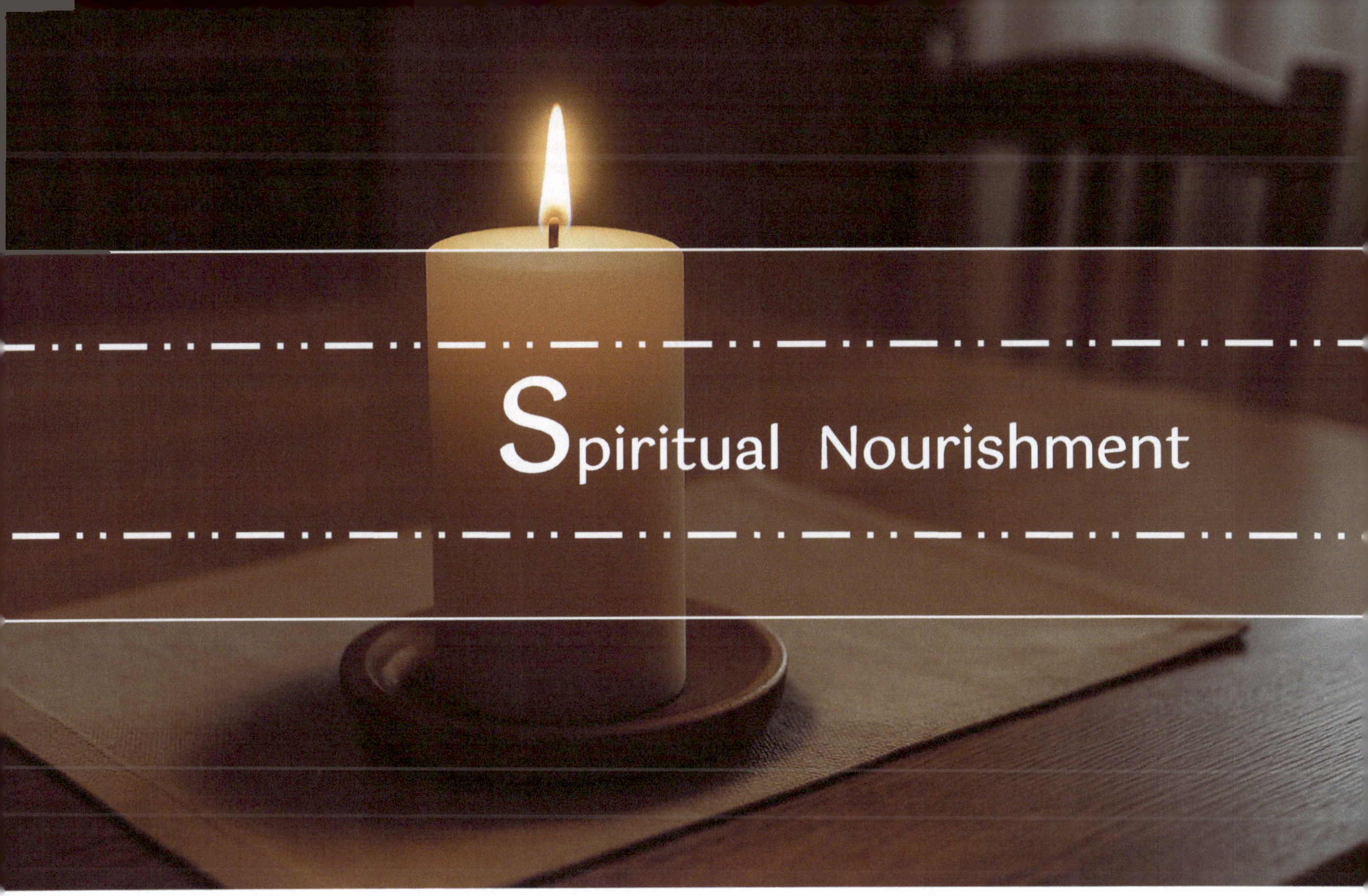

Spiritual Nourishment

When you are struggling, you may feel that you have been abandoned by God or any spiritual force that has power in this world. What I have been taught, though, is that these seasons of difficulty are intended not only to strengthen us and enrich our knowledge of ourselves and the world, they are opportunities for us to draw closer to the divine. Get to know Spirit on a personal level as you move through this season.

Thirst For Life

I know that what you are going through is not your fault. Life is unfair and challenging for everyone. Your health and circumstances are a product of your DNA, your upbringing, and a zillion variables that are beyond your control.

Still, you might be playing a role in your difficulties without realizing it. And now is when it might matter most.

It is so easy to get down when you are sick or have experienced a loss. It is completely understandable if you don't look forward to waking up, don't want to get out of bed, dread fulfilling your responsibilities, and can't get excited about anything. But the biggest problem is that your body is listening to you.

If you don't look forward to waking up, your body might decide to increase your fatigue. Don't want to get out of bed? Maybe some extra pain and stiffness can help keep you down. Dread your responsibilities? Brain fog, breathlessness, heart palpitations, nausea, whatever symptoms it is easiest for your body to create could be exacerbated by your thoughts.

Don't get me wrong. This doesn't always happen, and it's usually not how things start, but there are countless scientific studies and personal stories that prove that our attitudes make a difference.

One of the easiest, most important ways to communicate to your body that you want to heal and be healthy is to eat good food. Eating at all is a great start in communicating your desire to be alive. Eating good food is even better.

Take a moment during your meal to think about how the food tastes. Notice the texture, temperature, colors, everything you can. Does it bring up memories? Does it make you feel alive even if it doesn't make you happy?

Think about all of the miracles of sunlight, rain, earth, minerals, farmers, pollinators, transportation, electric refrigeration and stoves, and this humble cookbook. What a blessing that all of this came together so that you could have this food to sustain your life, heal your ills, make you stronger, and delight your senses.

Eat with gusto, and face life with passion. Celebrate being alive. Count your responsibilities like a list of blessings.

This is the true path to good health.

Strengthen Your Throat Chakra with Your Voice

The throat chakra comes into play when you are eating because it is the energy center located precisely where you swallow your food. For this reason, it has a large impact on your zest for life.

The throat chakra rules your expression of yourself. Obviously, it gives you voice and lets you speak your truth. In fact, every thing you do, every posture you take, every experience you accept is, in essence, expressing the unique nature of your being.

If you are having a hard time finding the will to eat, if you are sometimes unable to swallow food, if you just can't accept the bad thing that interrupted your plans, then pay attention to your throat chakra. It is hard at work enabling your soul to affect your physical body.

You can give some love to your throat chakra, and see if it helps change your experience of eating and your attitude toward life.

Start by doing some singing. This is really good for your Vagus nerve, too. Go for a walk in the woods where no one can hear you, and remember your favorite childhood songs. Sing in the shower. Join a choir. Hum while you do housework. Play a movie with a great soundtrack and sing along.

Other ways of nurturing your throat chakra include gently applying olive oil and massaging your throat and neck; wearing a blue crystal on a necklace chain; enjoying some mindful breathing; having an open conversation with a loved one; and getting a Reiki treatment and asking the practitioner to cleanse and open your throat chakra.

It will be interesting to discover how these practices affect your appetite and experience with food.

Meal Blessings from Around the World

Any words that you speak from your heart will bless your food, improve your attitude, and enhance the health-giving benefits of your meal. In case you have a hard time knowing just what to say, here are a variety of traditional prayers from around the world to give you inspiration.

Catholic Prayer: Bless Us, O Lord

Bless us, O Lord,
And these Thy gifts
Which we are about to receive
Through Thy bounty.
Through Christ our Lord, we pray.

From the Native American Iroquois Tradition

We return thanks to the corn, and to her sisters,
the beans and squashes, which give us life.
We return thanks to the bushes and trees,
which provide us with fruit.
We return thanks to the Great Spirit,
in who is embodied all goodness,
and who directs all things for the good of his children.

Christian Children's Prayer

Thank you, God, for the world so sweet,
Thank you God for the food we eat.
Thank you God for the birds that sing,
Thank you God for everything.

Meal Prayer adapted from Buddhist Teacher Thich Nhat Hanh

May the food we are eating make us aware of the
interconnections between Universe and us,
Earth and us, and all other living species and us.
Because each bite contains in itself
the life of Sun and Earth.
May we see the meaning and value of life from these
precious morsels of food.

Our Heavenly Father, Kind and Good

Our Heavenly Father, kind and good,
We thank Thee for our daily food.
Oh, may the strength it gives us be
Used every day in serving thee.

Moravian Dinner Prayer

Come, Lord Jesus, our guest to be
And bless these gifts
Bestowed by Thee.
And bless our loved ones everywhere,
And keep them in Your loving care.

Waldorf/Steiner Kindergarten Meal Blessing

Blessings on the blossom,
Blessings on the root
Blessings on the leaf and stem,
Blessings on the fruit.

Jewish Blessings

Blessed are You, Lord our God, Sovereign of the Universe, who brings forth bread from the earth.
Blessed are You, Lord our God, King of the universe, by Whose word all things came to be.

Hindu Prayer

Before grasping this grain,
let us consider in our minds
the reasons why
we should care for and safeguard this body.
This is my prayer, oh God:
May I be forever devoted at your feet,
offering body, mind, and wealth
to the service of truth in the world.

Sufi Meal Blessing

O Thou, the Sustainer of our bodies, hearts, and souls, bless all that we receive in thankfulness. Amen.

Celtic Prayer

God in our waking, God in our speaking,
God in our cooking, God in our eating,
God in our playing, God in our digesting,
God in our working, God in our Resting.

A Unitarian Blessing

Blessed be the Earth for giving birth to this food
Blessed be the Sun for nourishing it
Blessed be the Wind for carrying its seed
Blessed be the Rain for quenching its thirst.
Blessed be the hands that helped to grow this food,
To bring it to our tables
To nourish our minds, bodies, and spirits.
Blessed be our friends, our families, and our loved ones.
Blessed Be.

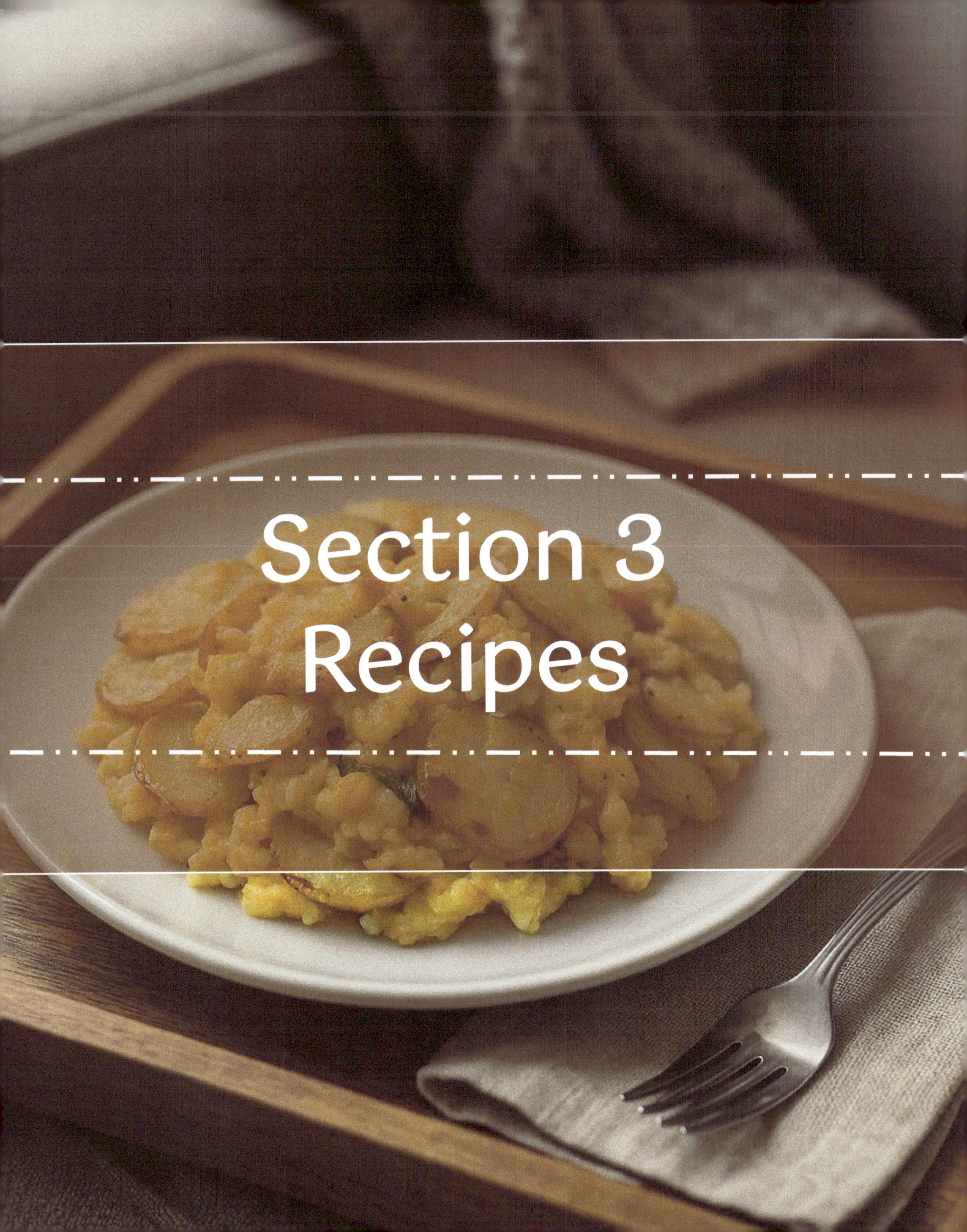

Section 3
Recipes

Gentle Starts

Breakfasts

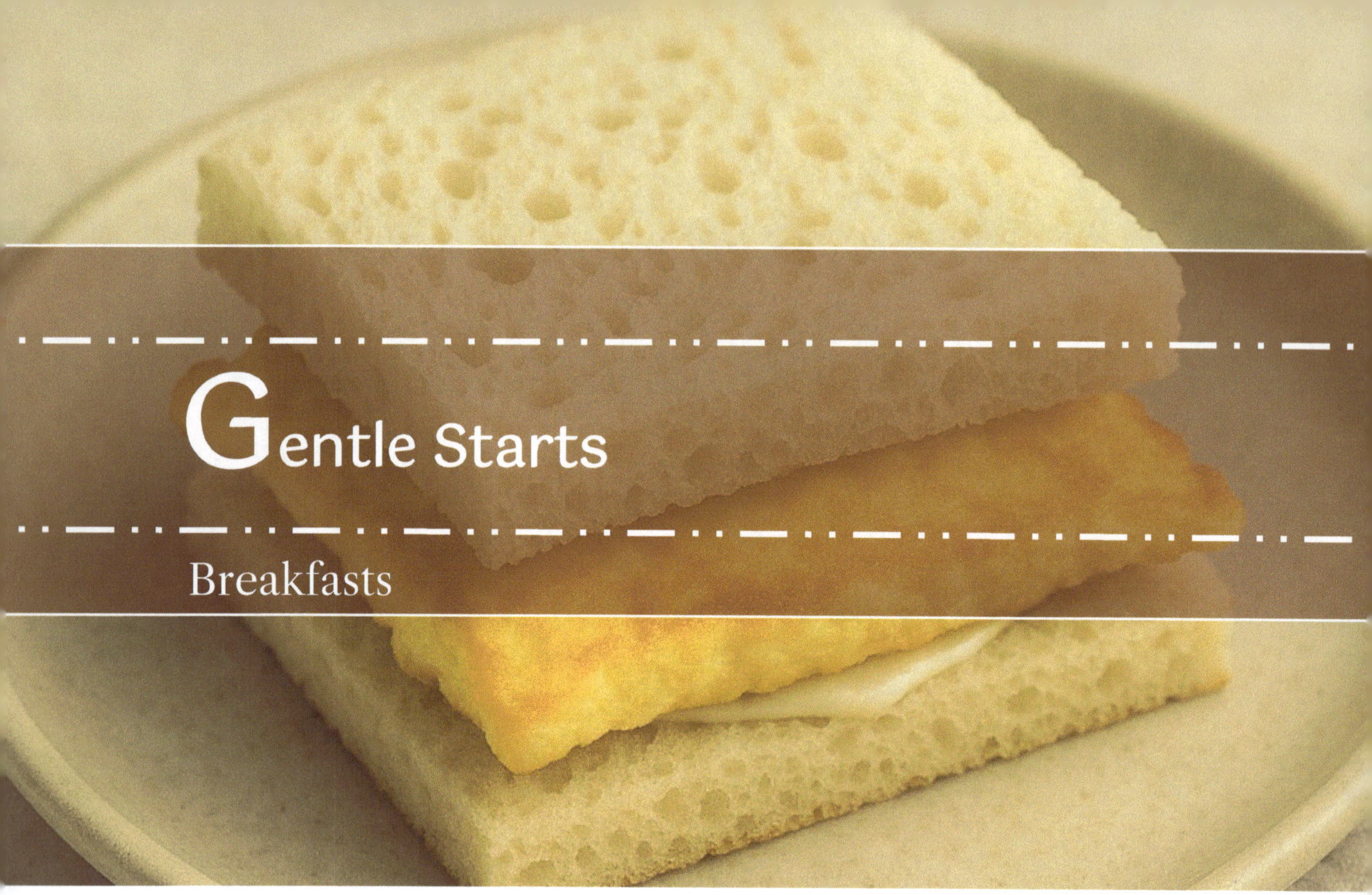

Fluffy Egg Sandwich

This is a soft, mild sandwich that can be a good source of protein when you're barely up to eating. It cooks up really fast with barely any work.

Time

5 minutes total

Servings

1 serving

Tools

Extra small skillet, preferred

Cereal bowl

Fork or whisk

Table knife

Ingredients

1 Tablespoon butter [14 g]

1 egg

2 pieces of soft bread

1 Tablespoon mayonnaise [15 g]

Directions

1. Melt **1 Tablespoon butter** in a small skillet over low heat.
2. While the butter is melting, crack **1 egg** into a bowl and whisk it until the yolk and white are well combined.
3. Once the butter is melted, swirl it around the pan and then pour the egg into the pan.
4. Wait until the bottom of the egg is solid but still soft and not brown; there will be liquid egg on top. Use a spatula to flip the egg, allowing the remaining liquid egg to go into the bottom of the pan.
5. While the egg is cooking, remove the crusts from **2 pieces of bread.**
6. Coat one side of each of the pieces of bread with **1 Tablespoon mayonnaise.**
7. The egg will puff up in a matter of seconds. Once it does, before it can begin to brown, remove the egg from the pan and place it on one piece of bread, with the other slice of bread on top, mayonnaise sides in.
8. Serve immediately.

Effortless Banana Bread

Banana Bread sounds like a home-baked treat that you would need to slave over, but it is very easy to make in a food processor and provides ready-made food for many days. After it cools, slice it and freeze it in zip baggies for future meals. Leftover banana bread toasted dark and coated with butter might be even better than fresh from the oven. Note that the recipe calls for overripe bananas, but if you have histamine issues, you may be better off using perfectly ripe fruit. If your bananas are getting ripe and you're not ready to bake, peel them and put them in the freezer in a baggie for later.

Time

1 hour 20 minutes total

Prep: 10 minutes   Bake: 1 hour

Rest and Cool: 10 minutes

Servings

12 servings

Tools

Food processor

9" x 5" bread pan

Ingredients

1 Tablespoon butter for coating pan [14 g]

3 overripe bananas (fresh or frozen)

2 cups flour [240 g]

1 teaspoon baking soda [6 g]

1 cup real maple syrup or honey [312 g]

1 egg

1/2 teaspoon salt [3 g]

1/4 cup butter, softened or melted [57 g]

1/2 cup pecans (or other nuts, optional) [54 g]

Directions

1. **Butter** the bottom and sides of a 9"x5" bread pan.
2. Mash **3 bananas** in a food processor on high until smooth.

3. Add **1 teaspoon baking soda**, **1 cup maple syrup, 1 egg, 1/2 teaspoon salt,** and **1/4 cup butter**. Mix on low until ingredients are combined.
4. Add **2 cups flour**. Pulse food processor until ingredients are combined, but do not over mix.
5. Add **1/2 cup pecans**. Pulse food processor a couple times until the nuts are mixed in.
6. Bake at 350 degrees for 1 hour or until toothpick comes out clean.
7. Allow to rest and cool 10 minutes before slicing. It can be removed from the pan and sliced on a cutting board or sliced in the pan.

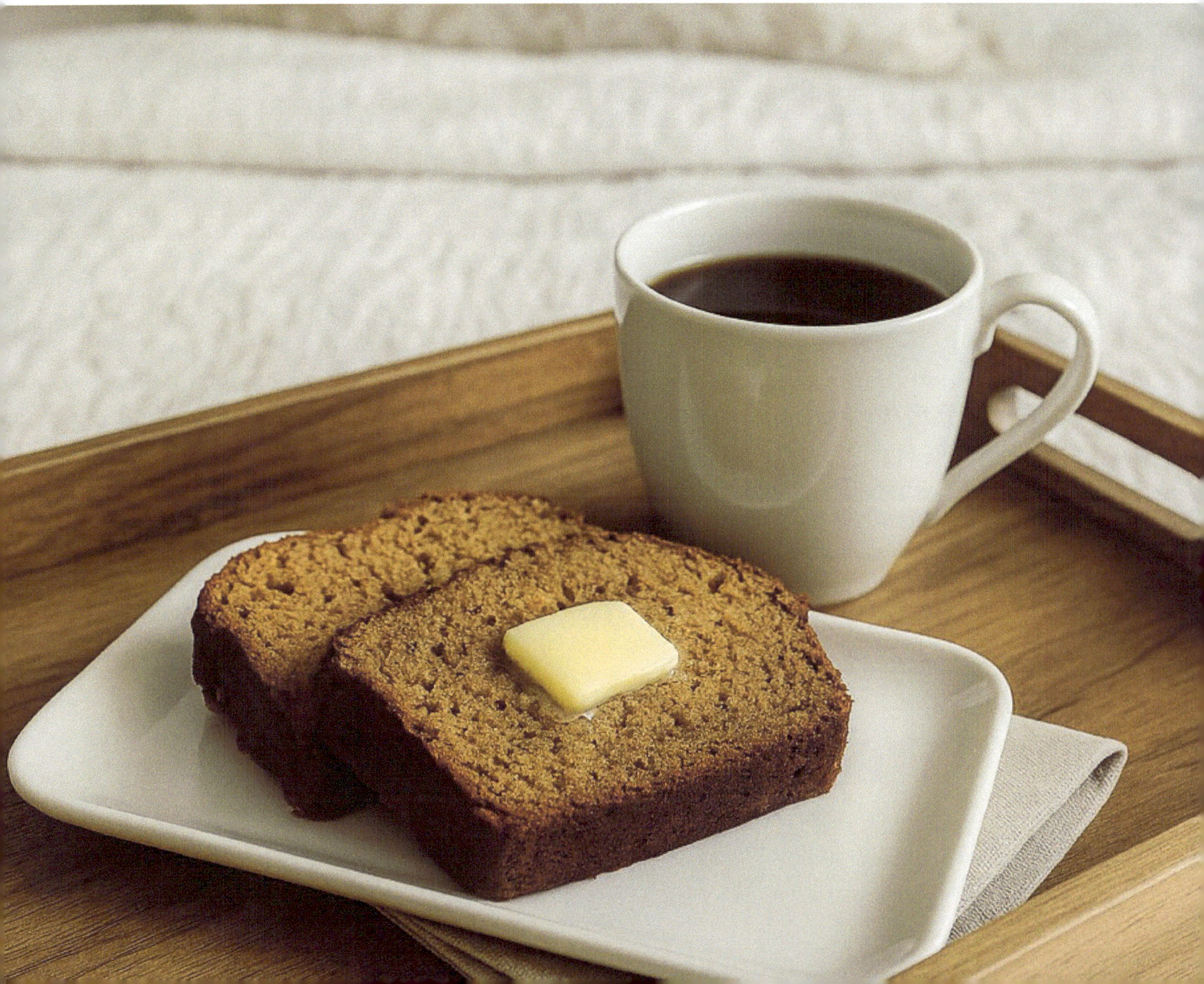

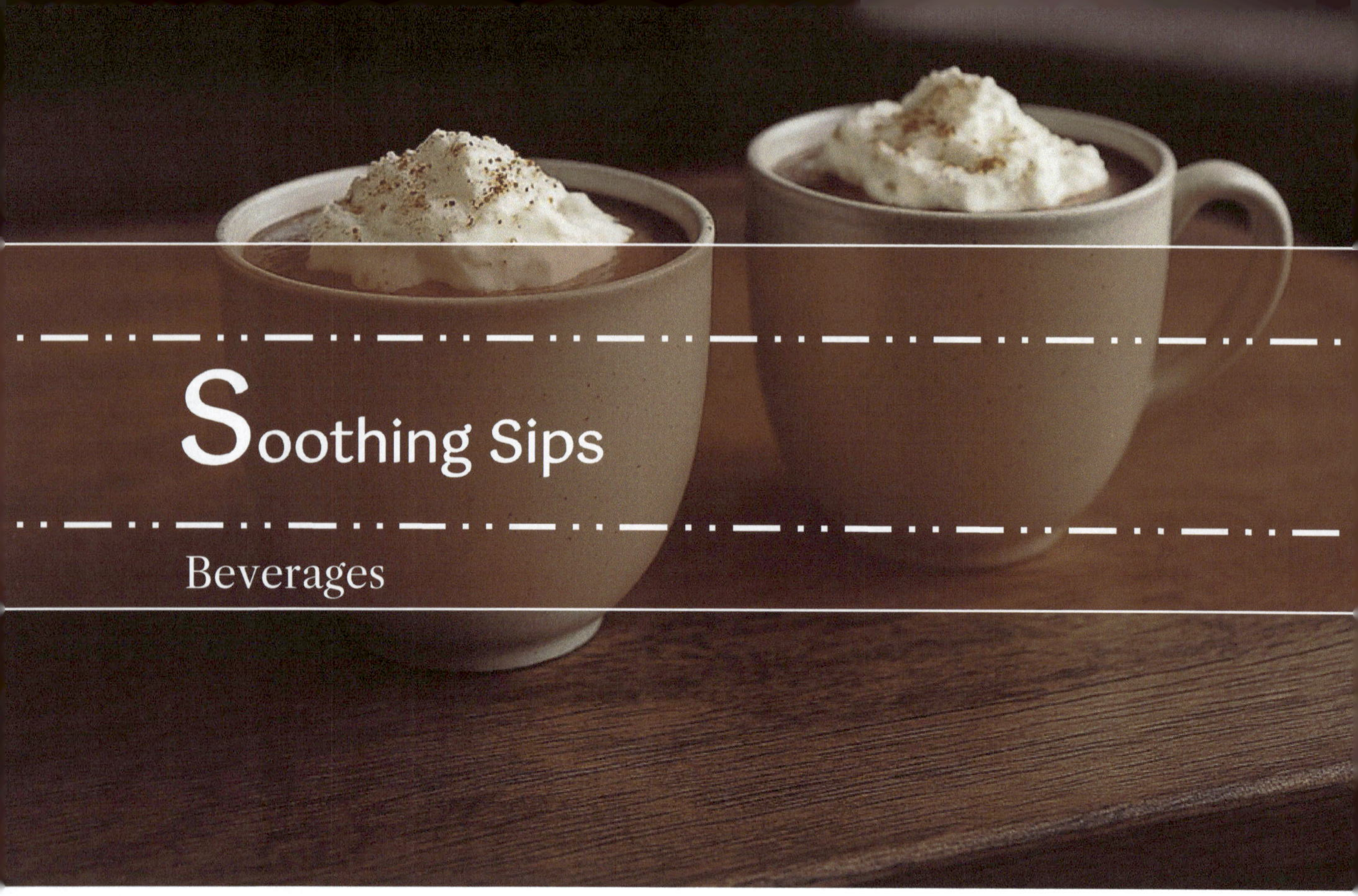

Soothing Sips

Beverages

Healing Spice Cocoa

This is one of the most delicious beverages in existence, according to my family, but the best part of it is that it can stave off a cold if you drink it just as soon as you feel the tickle of a sore throat starting. This beverage is also very good for warming you up if you are outside in the wintertime. It seems like a decadent treat, but every ingredient is health-giving. Cayenne is a more powerful medicine than paprika, but it is spicier.

Time

10 minutes

Servings

1 serving

Tools

Pot

Whisk (or spoon or fork)

Ingredients

1 cup whole milk, raw preferred [227 g]

1 heaping Tablespoon unsweetened cocoa powder [10 g]

1-2 Tablespoon real maple syrup [20-40 g]

1/4 teaspoon ground cinnamon [1 g]

1/4 teaspoon ground chili powder [1 g]

1/8 teaspoon ground cayenne pepper or paprika [0.5 g]

Dash of salt

Whipped cream for topping (optional)

Directions

1. In a small pot, heat **1 cup milk** over medium-high heat, whisking almost constantly. Use an electric pot stirrer, if needed.
2. When steam and a lot of small bubbles begin to appear on top of the milk, add in **1 generous Tablespoon cocoa powder**. Continue whisking until the cocoa has melted and is well combined.
3. Add **1-2 Tablespoons maple syrup, 1/4 teaspoon cinnamon, 1/4 teaspoon chili powder, dash of salt**, and **⅛ teaspoon cayenne or paprika**.
4. Serve immediately. You can top it with real **whipped cream** if desired.

Bright Berry Slushie

These are such a delightful treat, you won't believe how much tastier they are than the slushies you can buy (that are full of sugar and artificial colors and flavors). And yet, they're unbelievably easy to make and extremely good for you. A refreshing treat for a hot summer day!

Time

5 minutes

Servings

1 serving

Tools

Blender

Ingredients

1 handful of fresh, clean berries (strawberries are a clear favorite, but raspberries are close behind; frozen berries will work just as well as fresh)

2 handfuls of ice

1-2 teaspoons real maple syrup [5-10 g]

Directions

1. Place all ingredients in a blender: **berries, ice,** and **maple syrup**.
2. Blend until smooth, adding water if it is too thick.
3. Drink with a straw.

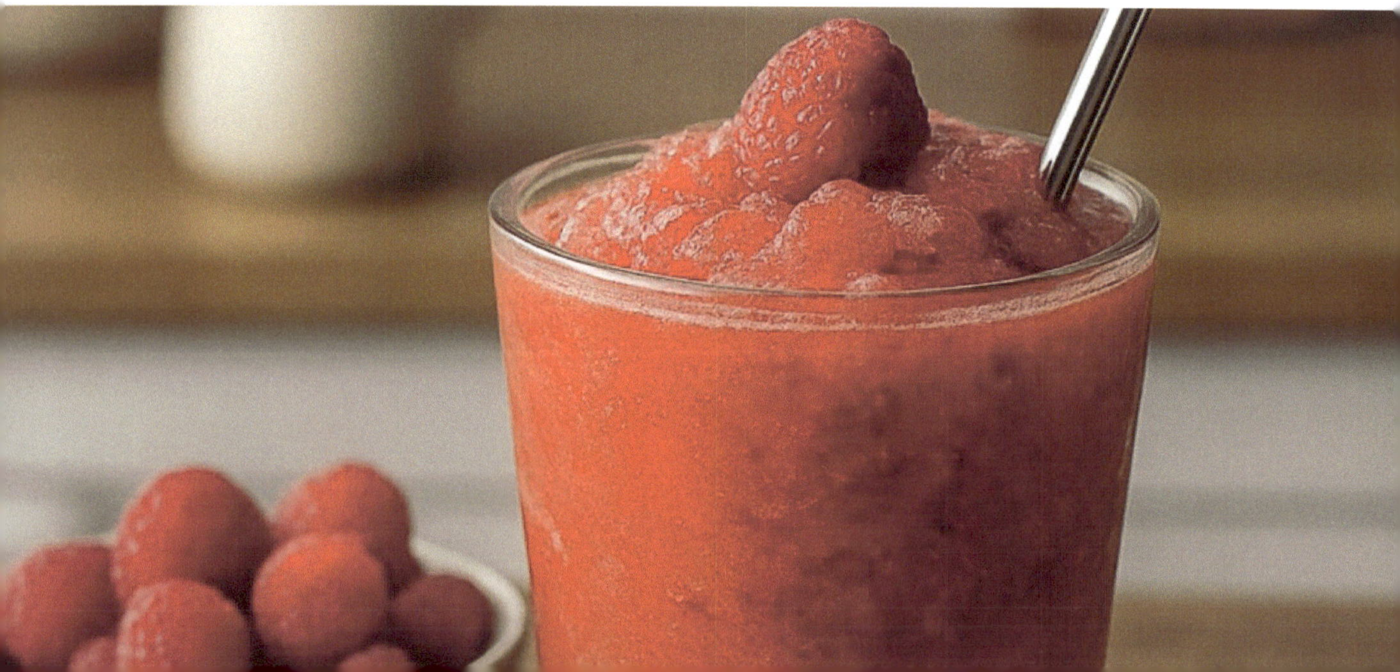

Warming Spiced Chai

This is inspired by the Indian beverage that is beloved in the Ayurveda tradition of health and wellness. It is warming and invigorating. Each of the spices contain healing constituents that are especially beneficial for improving circulation during the cold months. Use whole or ground spices.

Time

15 minutes

Servings

1 serving

Tools

Pot

Whisk (or spoon)

Strainer

Ingredients

1 teaspoon loose-leaf black tea (oolong, English breakfast, or any variety is suitable) [2 g]

1 cup water [227 g]

1 cup raw whole milk [227 g]

1/2 teaspoon cinnamon [2 g]

1/4 teaspoon ginger [1 g]

1/4 teaspoon cloves [1 g]

1/4 teaspoon cardamom [1 g]

Dash of black pepper

1-2 Tablespoons maple syrup or honey [20-40 g]

Directions

1. Put **1 teaspoon tea, 1 cup water, 1 cup milk, and all of the spices: 1/2 teaspoon cinnamon, 1/4 teaspoon ginger, and 1/4 teaspoon cardamom**, and **a dash of black pepper** into a pot.
2. Heat over medium-high heat, whisking constantly, until the milk begins to froth.
3. Pour through a strainer into a large mug, and discard leaves and spices.
4. Add **maple syrup** to taste, and serve hot.

Banana Cloud Shake

It tastes like a milkshake, sweet and delicious, but it contains no sugar! This is a hearty beverage that can settle my stomach quickly when it is upset. It is also a go-to breakfast when I am worried that I can't stomach anything. It is a very nice accompaniment to a warm piece of toast with peanut butter on it.

Time

5 minutes

Servings

1 serving

Tools

Blender

Small spoon such as a measuring spoon

Ingredients

1 banana (the riper the better)

1 cup milk [227 g]

Directions

1. Peel **1 banana** and slice it lengthwise down the middle. Use a small spoon to scoop the seeds out and discard them.
2. Blend the banana and **1 cup milk** very well in a blender or with an immersion blender. It will froth up quite a lot.
3. Drink it immediately, as it will deflate quickly. (Also, rinse the glass after drinking so that the milkshake won't stick and be difficult to clean.)

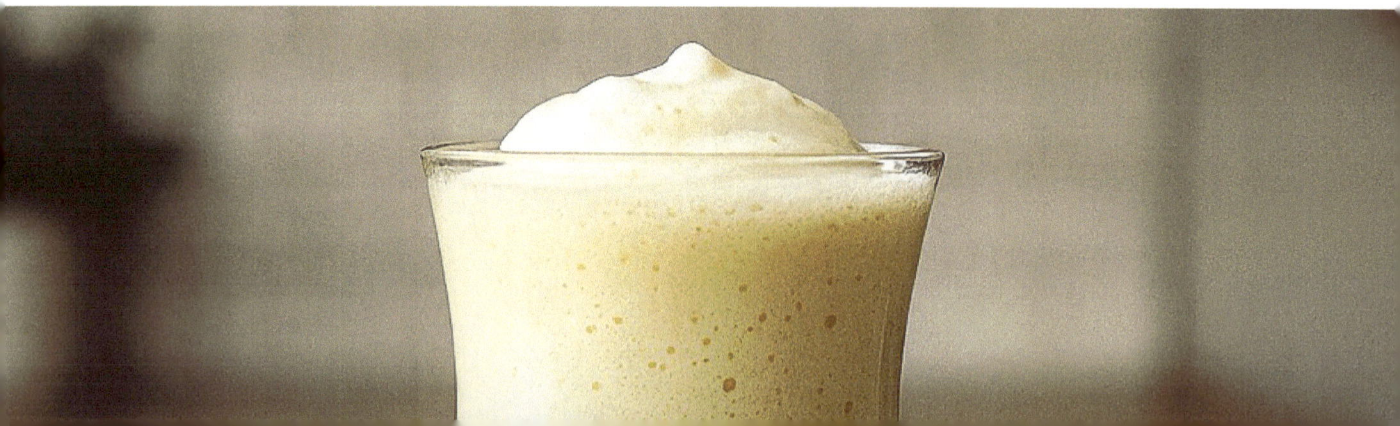

Quick Cinnamon Protein Nog

This is a healthy, high-protein, quick breakfast, better for you than protein powders. It is actually a simplified version of a holiday eggnog. Many people think they don't like eggnog because they have only had storebought versions. This is very tasty! For breakfast, I like it served with buttered toast.

Time

5 minutes

Servings

1 serving

Tools

Blender

Ingredients

1 raw egg (only use an egg from a trusted local farmer)

1 cup milk [227 g]

1 Tablespoon real maple syrup [20 g]

1/4 teaspoon vanilla extract (alcohol-free preferred, optional) [1 g]

1/4 teaspoon ground cinnamon (optional) [1 g]

1/8 teaspoon nutmeg (optional) [.5 g]

Directions

1. Put all ingredients into a blender: **1 egg, 1 cup milk, 1 Tablespoon syrup, 1/4 teaspoon vanilla, 1/4 teaspoon cinnamon,** and **1/8 teaspoon nutmeg**. (The spices can be withheld and sprinkled on top if you prefer.)
2. Blend until well mixed and frothy.
3. Serve immediately.

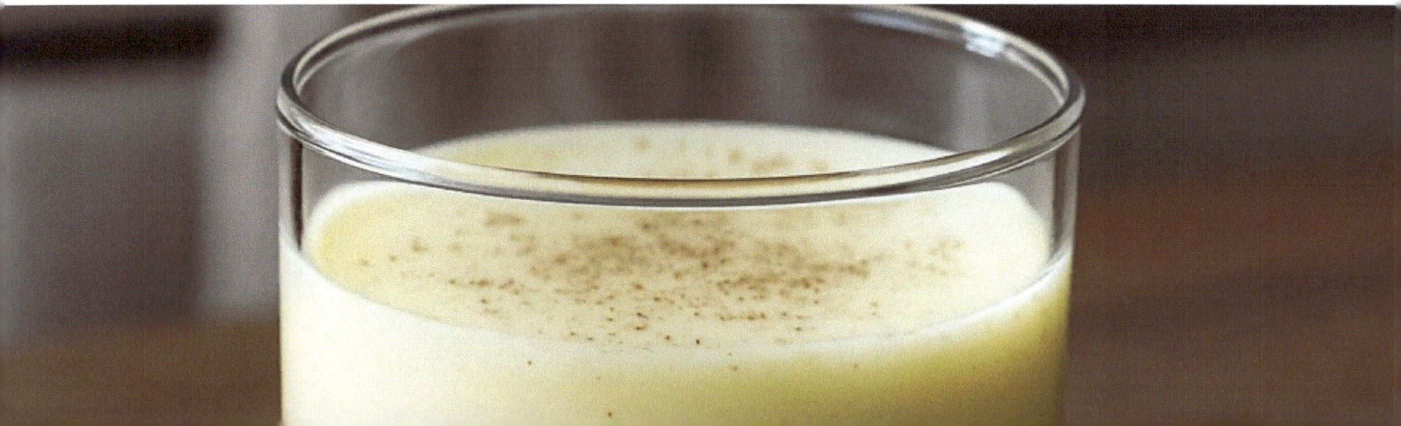

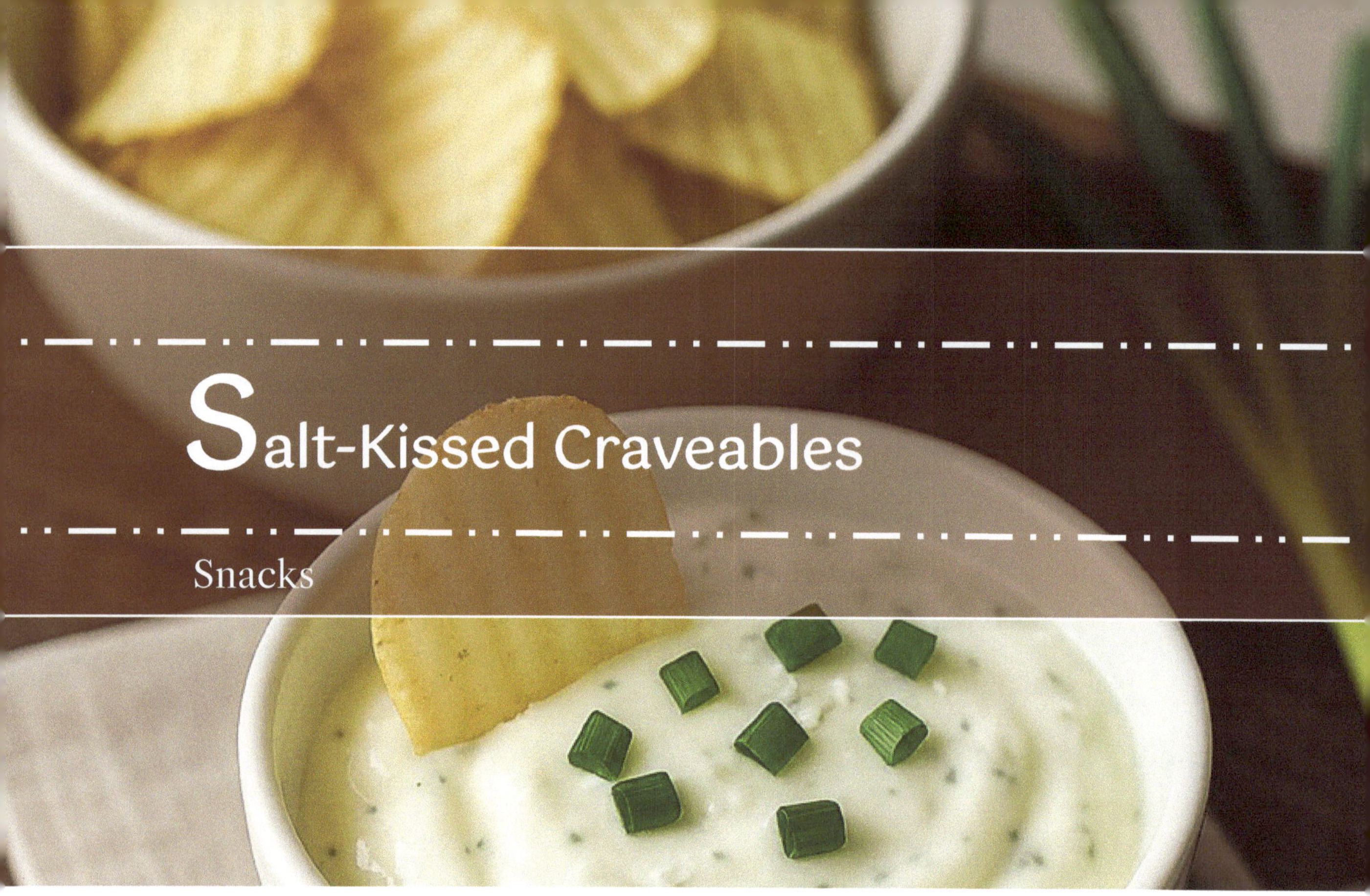

Salt-Kissed Craveables

Snacks

Spring Tonic Dip

This dip is delicious any time of year, if you come across fresh green onions, but it is especially helpful in the springtime when the green onions are at their best. It is also delicious made with garlic scapes instead of green onions.

Time

5 minutes

Servings

4 servings

Tools

Small bowl

Knife

Cutting board

Ingredients

1 bunch of green onions (and/or garlic scapes), diced

1 cup of sour cream [227 g]

1/2 teaspoon salt [3 g]

Potato chips or celery sticks (or both)

Directions

1. Combine **1 bunch of diced green onions**, **1 cup of sour cream,** and **1/2 teaspoon salt** in a bowl, and stir with a spoon.
2. Serve with plain salted **potato chips or celery sticks**.
3. The dip will get better if you let it sit in the fridge for at least an hour in order for the flavors to blend, but it is already delicious as soon as it is mixed.

Buttery Succotash

This old traditional side dish makes for a nice salty snack. Frozen vegetables are low in histamine, plus this recipe provides sweetness, protein, fat, vitamins, and salt, a nutritionally complete choice!

Time

5 minutes

Servings

1 serving

Tools

Small pot

Spoon

Ingredients

1/2 cup frozen sweet corn [85 g]

1/2 cup frozen lima beans [83 g]

1-2 Tablespoons butter [14-28 g]

Salt, to taste

Directions

1. Put **1/2 cup sweet corn and 1/2 cup lima beans** into a small pot over medium-low heat. Heat until warmed through, stirring occasionally.
2. Add **1 Tablespoon butter** or more, and stir until it is melted. **Salt** to taste and serve immediately.

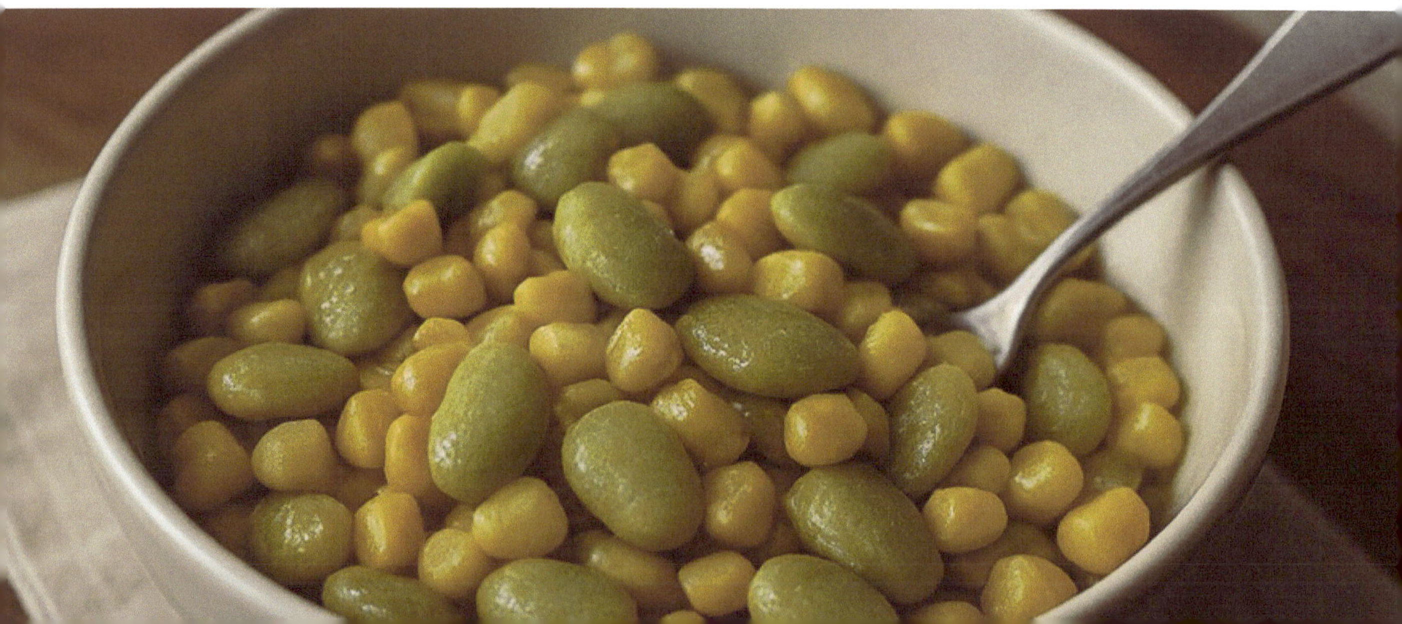

Sunny Avocado Snack

Once you try this snack, you will start craving it when your body needs the fats, vitamin C, electrolytes, and salt it offers. It is surprising that such a simple dish can be so flavorful. I sometimes like to eat tortilla chips on the side.

Time

5 minutes

Servings

1 serving

Tools

Small bowl

Knife

Ingredients

1 ripe avocado

1/2-1 lemon

Salt, to taste

Directions

1. Cut **1 avocado** in half, remove the pit and skin. Place the two avocado halves in the bowl.
2. Cut **1 lemon**, and catching the seeds in your hand or a strainer, squeeze lemon juice over the avocado.
3. **Salt** liberally, and serve.

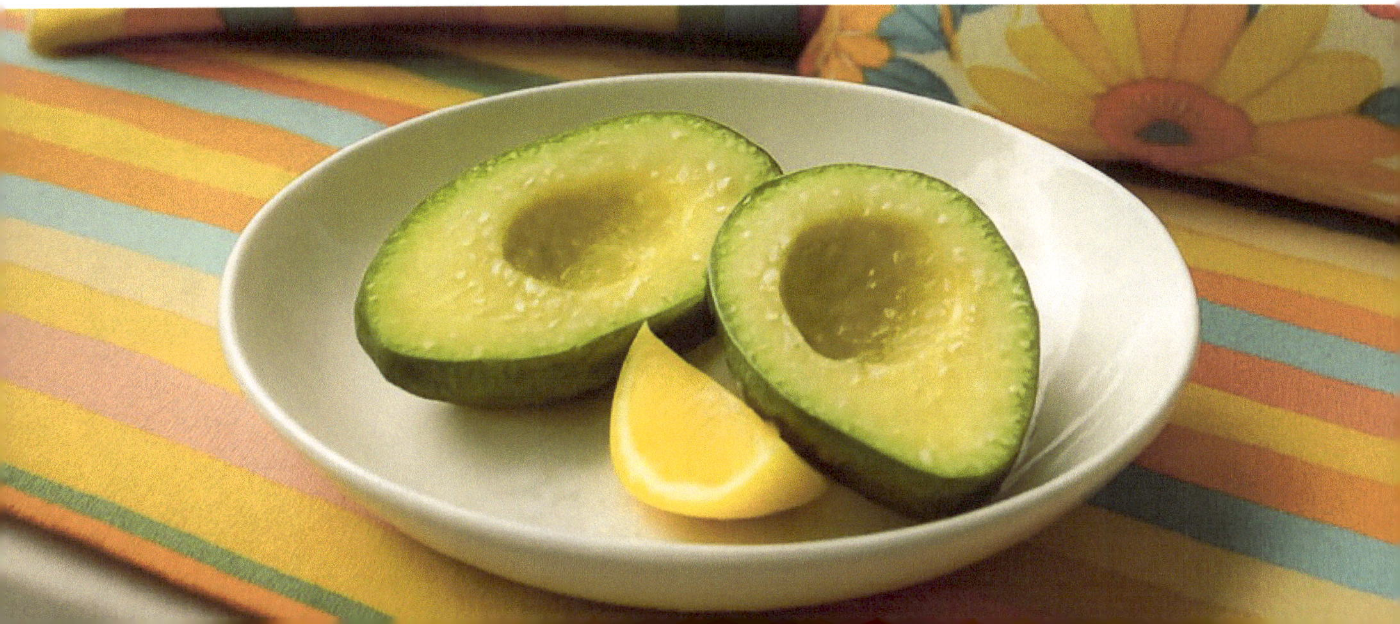

Curry Tuna Personal Party Dip

This makes for a delicious appetizer at a party, served with crackers. Put it on bread for a not-your-usual tuna sandwich. Or, make an elegant luncheon salad by cutting a tomato into quarters on top of a bed of lettuce, putting a scoop of Curry Tuna Personal Party Dip in the center, and topping it with halved red grapes. You can also shake an extra sprinkling of curry powder on top for an extra punch of flavor.

Time

5 minutes

Servings

2 servings

Tools

Small bowl

Spoons

Ingredients

1 can tuna [142 g]

1 Tablespoon mayonnaise [14 g]

1 Tablespoon sweet pickle relish [15 g]

1/2 teaspoon curry powder [2 g]

Directions

1. Put **1 can tuna, 1 Tablespoon mayonnaise, 1 Tablespoon sweet pickle relish,** and **1/2 teaspoon curry powder** in a bowl. Mix to combine. Serve in a bowl with a fork or as described above.

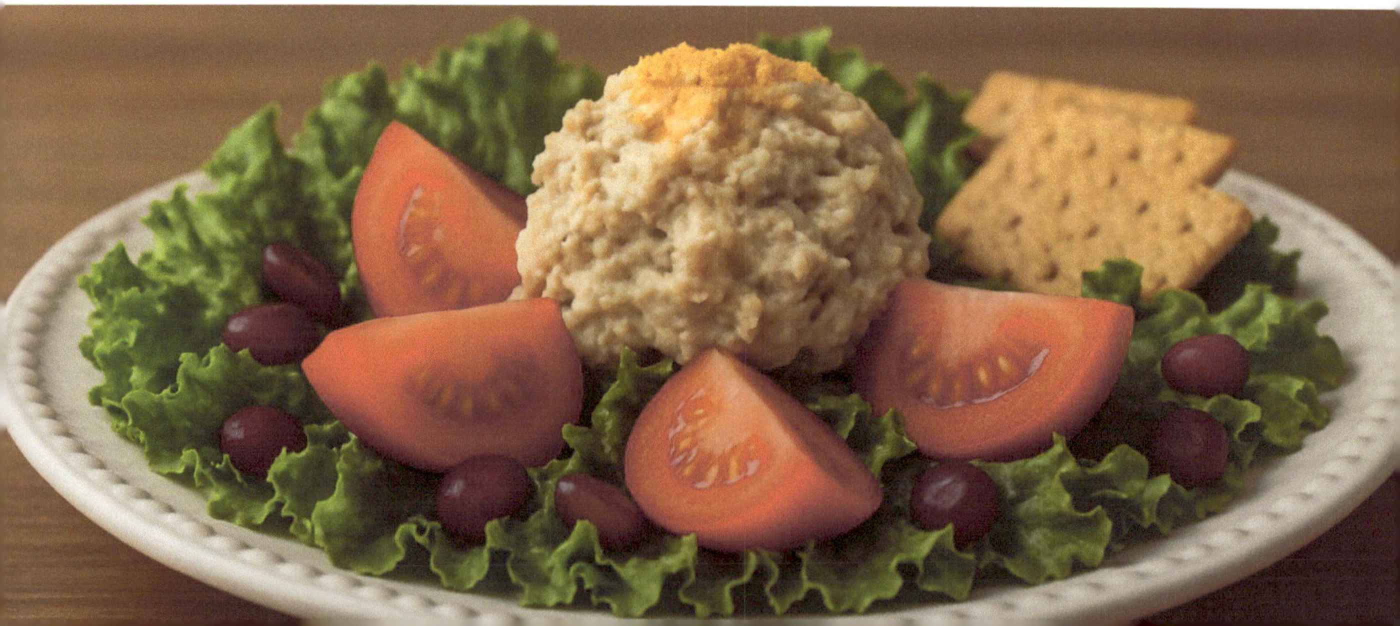

Nutritional Popcorn

Microwave popcorn will never compare to popcorn made on the stovetop. It requires no fancy tools and very little time, but the taste and nutritional content are exceptional. Make sure to choose an organic popcorn, and even better, an heirloom variety. Nutritional yeast is a super food, but be aware that some people with MCAS will react to nutritional yeast. Try to find a brand that is not fortified and has no added ingredients.

Time

10 minutes

Servings

1 serving

Tools

Medium pot with handle
Small pot with handle

Ingredients

2 Tablespoons butter [28 g]

1 Tablespoon olive oil [14 g]

2 Tablespoons popcorn kernels [30 g]

Nutritional yeast, to taste

Salt, to taste

Directions

1. Put **2 Tablespoons butter** into a small pot and melt on low heat.
2. While the butter is melting, put **1 Tablespoon olive oil** and **2 popcorn kernels** into a medium pot. Put the lid on, and heat over medium-high heat.
3. When the kernels pop, pour in **2 Tablespoons popcorn kernels**. Shake the pot to coat the kernels.
4. Allow the corn to pop over medium-high heat, shaking the pot occasionally. When the popping slows to less than 1 pop in 3 seconds, pour the popped corn into a bowl.
5. Drizzle the melted butter over the popcorn, sprinkle on **nutritional yeast** and **salt**, to taste.

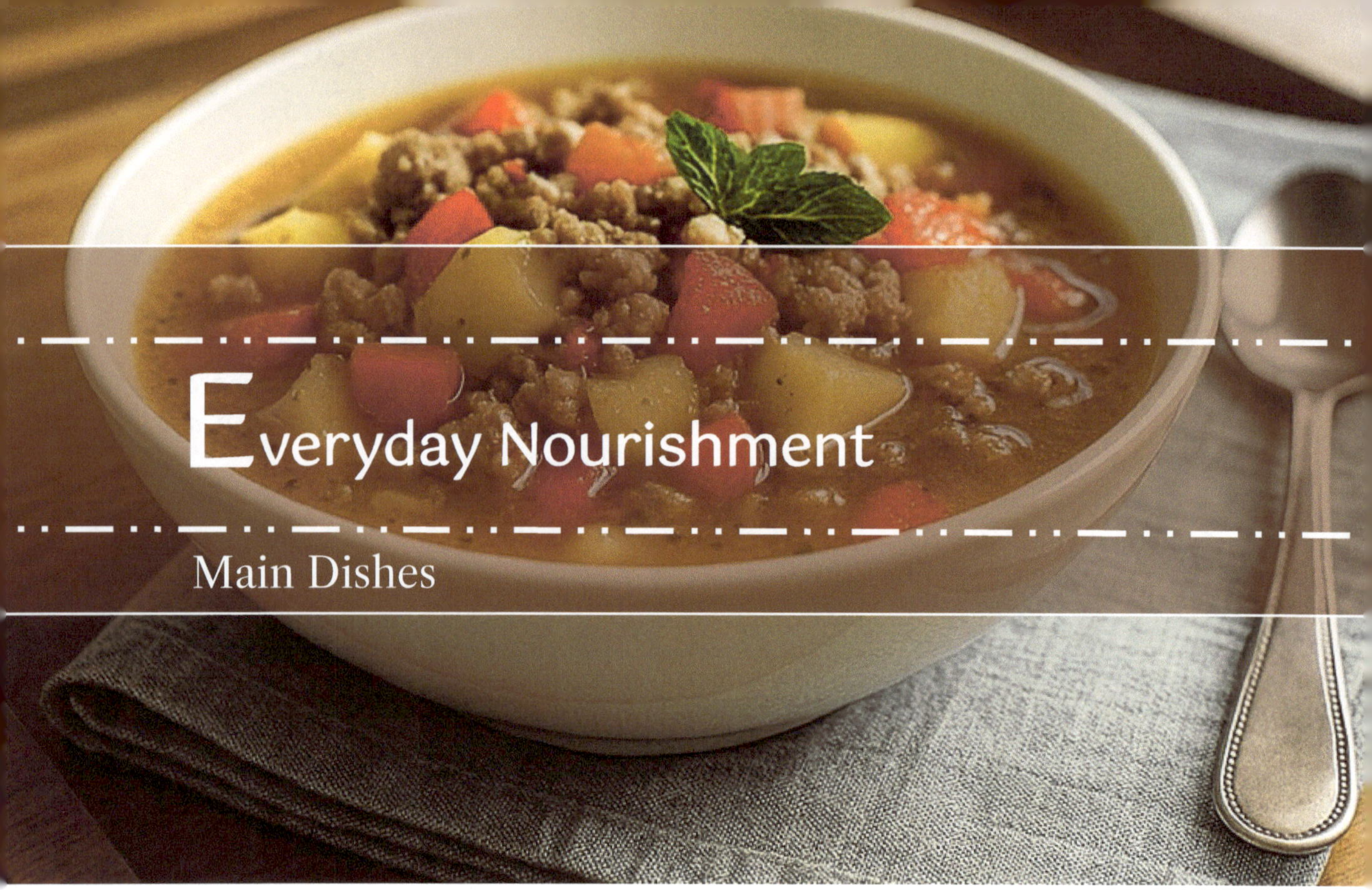

Italian Sausage Skillet

This recipe does require some chopping, but not a lot, and it is very simple but hearty and nourishing. If you are unable to find ground sausage, use links, discarding the skins. Russett or Golden potatoes are delicious in this recipe. The bell pepper can be red, orange, or yellow.

Time

30 minutes total

Active: 15 minutes

Cook: 15 minutes

Servings

8 servings

Tools

Knife

Cutting board

Skillet

Large spoon

Ingredients

1 pound ground mild Italian sausage [454 g]

3 potatoes, diced

1 red bell pepper, diced

1 teaspoon salt [6 g]

1/2 teaspoon dried oregano [2 g]

1 cup bone broth [240 g]

Red pepper flakes for sprinkling on top (optional)

Directions

1. Cook **1 pound ground mild Italian sausage** in a skillet over medium heat, breaking it into crumbled pieces, and stirring so that it browns evenly.
2. While the meat is cooking, dice the **3 potatoes** and **1 bell pepper**.
3. Once the meat is evenly browned, add the diced potatoes and bell pepper, **1 teaspoon salt, 1/2 teaspoon oregano**, and **1 cup bone broth**. If the liquid does not nearly cover the mixture, add a little bit more broth or water until it does.
4. Turn the heat up to bring the liquid to a gentle boil, then turn the heat to low. Put on the lid, and simmer gently for about 15 minutes, until the potatoes are soft.
5. Stir and then serve warm, adding **red pepper flakes** to each serving as desired.

Tender Pot Chicken

This is the easiest way to cook chicken and get it really tender. It makes a good main dish with any simple sides, or you can use it to make sandwiches, quesadillas, and some of the other recipes in this book. Chicken breasts will work for this recipe, but thighs cost less than breasts, tend to cook more evenly, and have more flavor.

Time

25 minutes total

Active: 5 minutes

Cook: 20 minutes

Servings

4 servings

Tools

Medium pot with lid

Tongs

Ingredients

1 pound chicken thighs, bones removed; skin is optional [454 g]

2 Tablespoons fat for the pan (bacon grease preferred) [26 g]

Salt and pepper to taste

Seasoning herbs, such as thyme or oregano (optional)

Directions

1. If the **1 pound chicken** has been cut so that it will lay very flat, you do not need to do anything to it, but if it is thick or has uneven thickness, you can either butterfly it, cut it into thinner strips, or put a piece of parchment paper over it and flatten it with a rolling pin.
2. Put **2 Tablespoons fat** in the pan and melt over medium high heat.
3. Sprinkle **salt, pepper,** and **seasoning herbs** onto one side of 1 pound of chicken.
4. Place the chicken in the melted fat so that the meat is flat. Season the top side of the chicken with salt, pepper, and herbs.
5. Cook until the meat releases easily from the pan, about 3 minutes, and then use tongs to flip it.

6. Put a lid on the pan and lower the heat to medium-low. Cook for 10 minutes.
7. Remove the pan from the heat but keep the lid on. Allow to sit for 10 minutes.
8. Serve warm or use in another recipe.

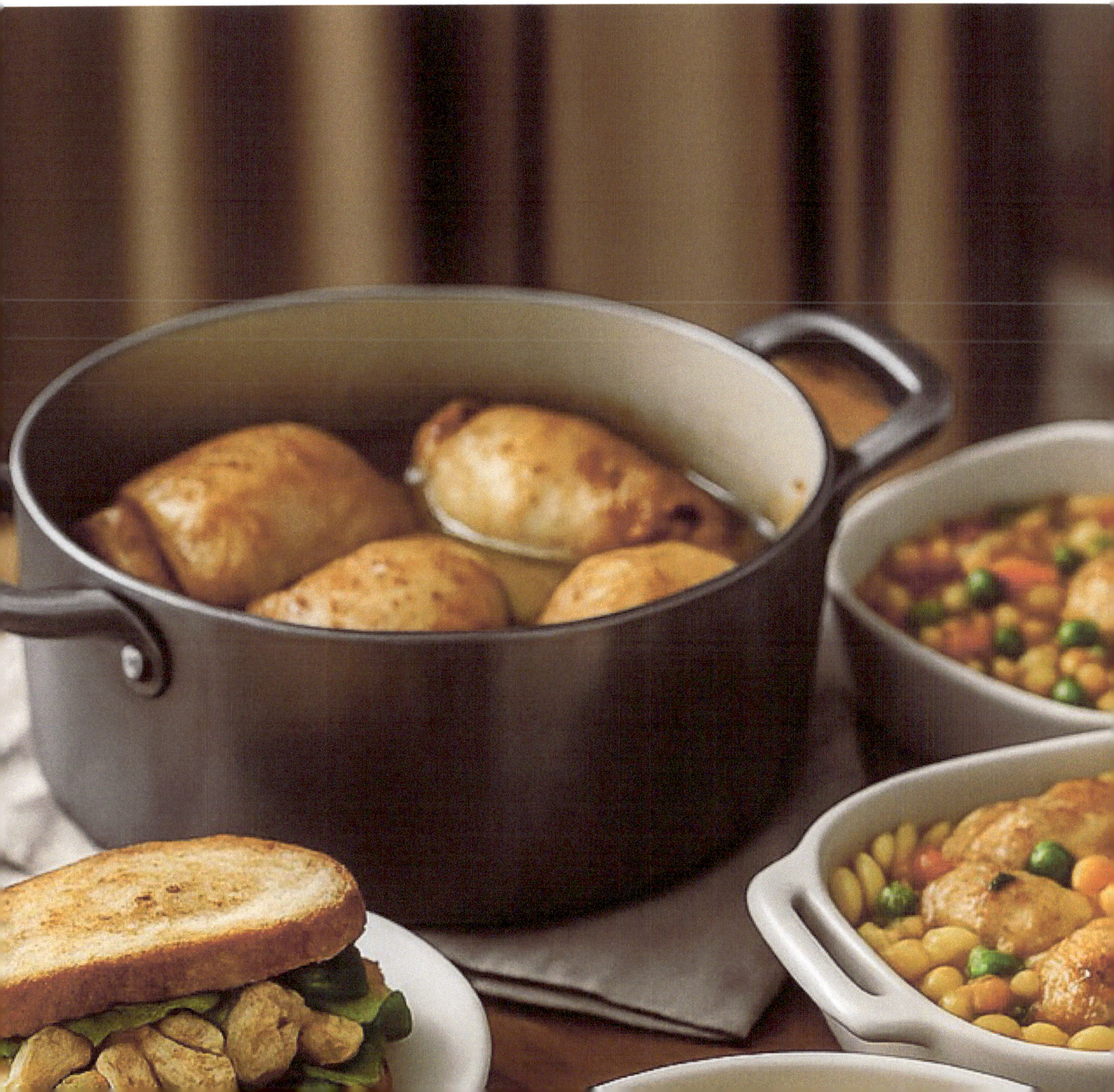

Propose to Me Pasta

This recipe is based on a popular dish called Marry Me Chicken – it's so good, if you cook it for your boyfriend, he'll want to marry you. That was true with mine! I have simplified the cooking process, reduced the ingredients, and put it on pasta to make it an easy recipe that is filling and delicious. Be aware that sundried tomatoes could be high histamine.

Time

40 minutes total

Active: 10 minutes

Cook: 30 minutes

Servings

6 servings

Tools

Skillet

Large spoon

Pot

Strainer

Ingredients

1 8-ounce jar (approximately) sliced sundried tomatoes in olive oil [240 g]

1 pound chicken thighs [454 g]

1/2 pound pasta (angel hair or corkscrew preferred) [227 g]

1 teaspoon salt [6 g]

1/2 teaspoon thyme [1 g]

3/4 cup bone broth [180 g]

1/2 cup heavy whipping cream [120 g]

Red pepper flakes to taste (optional)

Directions

1. Pour the oil only from **1 8-ounce jar of sundried tomatoes** into a skillet, reserving the tomatoes for later. Heat the oil very briefly over medium high heat. Add **1 pound chicken thighs,** spread out in the skillet. Cook for about 8 minutes on each side.
2. While the chicken is cooking, in a separate pot, cook **1/2 pound pasta** according to package directions.

3. When chicken is almost cooked through, add the **sundried tomatoes, 1 teaspoon salt, 1/2 teaspoon thyme,** and **3/4 cup bone broth** to the pan. Stir and bring to a simmer. Simmer for about 15 minutes, stirring occasionally. You can use the edge of the large spoon to cut the chicken into pieces, which will make it easier to serve and give you the opportunity to assure that it is cooked through.
4. When the chicken is cooked, add **1/2 cup heavy whipping cream** and stir.
5. To serve, put a serving of pasta in a dinner bowl. Spoon some of the sauce from the pan onto the pasta, and stir the pasta with a fork to coat it with the sauce. Then top it with the chicken and sundried tomatoes. Sprinkle with **red pepper flakes** if desired.

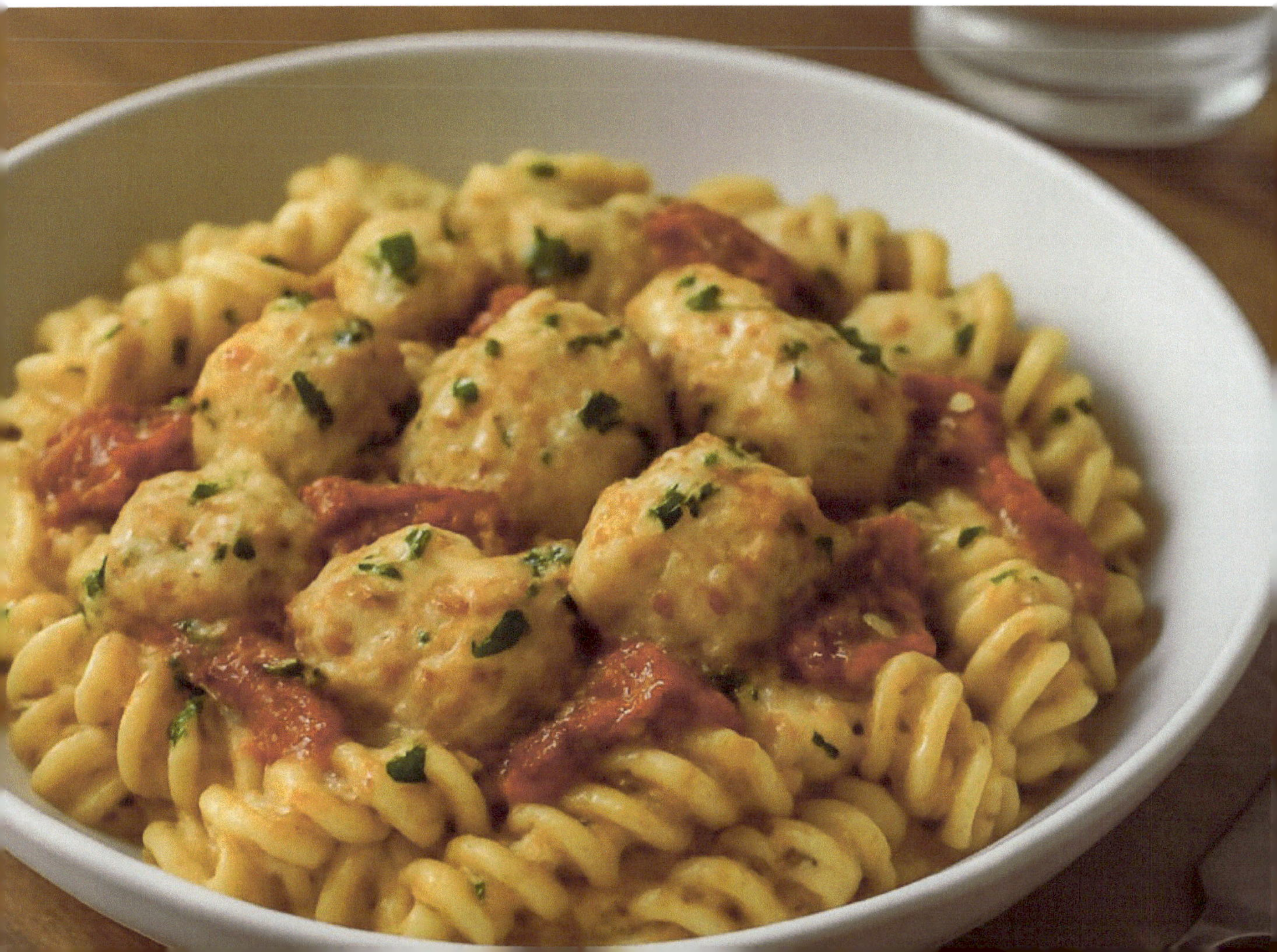

One-Skillet Spanish Rice

This is an ideal meal to cook when you have leftover rice, and it reduces the amount of work you have to do at once. White, brown, wild, basmati, or any kind will do. However, you can make fresh rice, and it will be just as good. For the chicken, you can prepare it fresh or use Tender Pot Chicken. The thighs can be kept whole or cut into 1/2-inch pieces, either before or after cooking. Pre-chopped frozen vegetables make it easy to prepare. The rich flavor of the paprika and other spices indicates it is chock full of nutrients.

Time

30-45 minutes total

Servings

4 servings

Tools

Skillet

Knife

Cutting board

Large spoon

Optional: medium pot with lid, spatula or tongs

Ingredients

1-2 Tablespoons fat for the pan]13-26 g]

1 pound cooked chicken [454 g]

1 red bell pepper, diced

1 cup frozen mixed veggies (carrots, green beans, and corn; fresh, chopped veggies would work, too) [135 g]

3 teaspoons ground paprika [6 g]

2 teaspoons salt [12 g]

1/4 teaspoon oregano [.5 g]

3/4 teaspoon ground cumin [2.25 g]

3/4 teaspoon ground coriander [2.25 g]

2 cups broth [480 g]

1 cup cooked rice, more or less [200 g]

Directions

1. If you are using fresh instead of leftover **rice**, prepare it according to package directions so that you have 1 cup once it is cooked.
2. If you are cooking **1 pound fresh chicken thighs**, heat **2 Tablespoon fat** in pan over medium heat.
3. Cook chicken for 5-8 minutes on each side, until cooked through.
4. Add **1 diced pepper, 1 cup frozen veggies, 3 teaspoons paprika, 2 teaspoons salt, 1/4 teaspoon oregano, 1/4 teaspoon cumin, 1/4 teaspoon coriander**, and **2 cups broth** to pan; if you are using **precooked chicken**, add it and the **fat** now.
5. Cook over medium heat for about 20 minutes, until the vegetables are as tender as you like them and everything is heated through.
6. Stir in **cooked rice**, and cook, stirring occasionally, about 3 minutes, until rice is refreshed, warm, and soft.

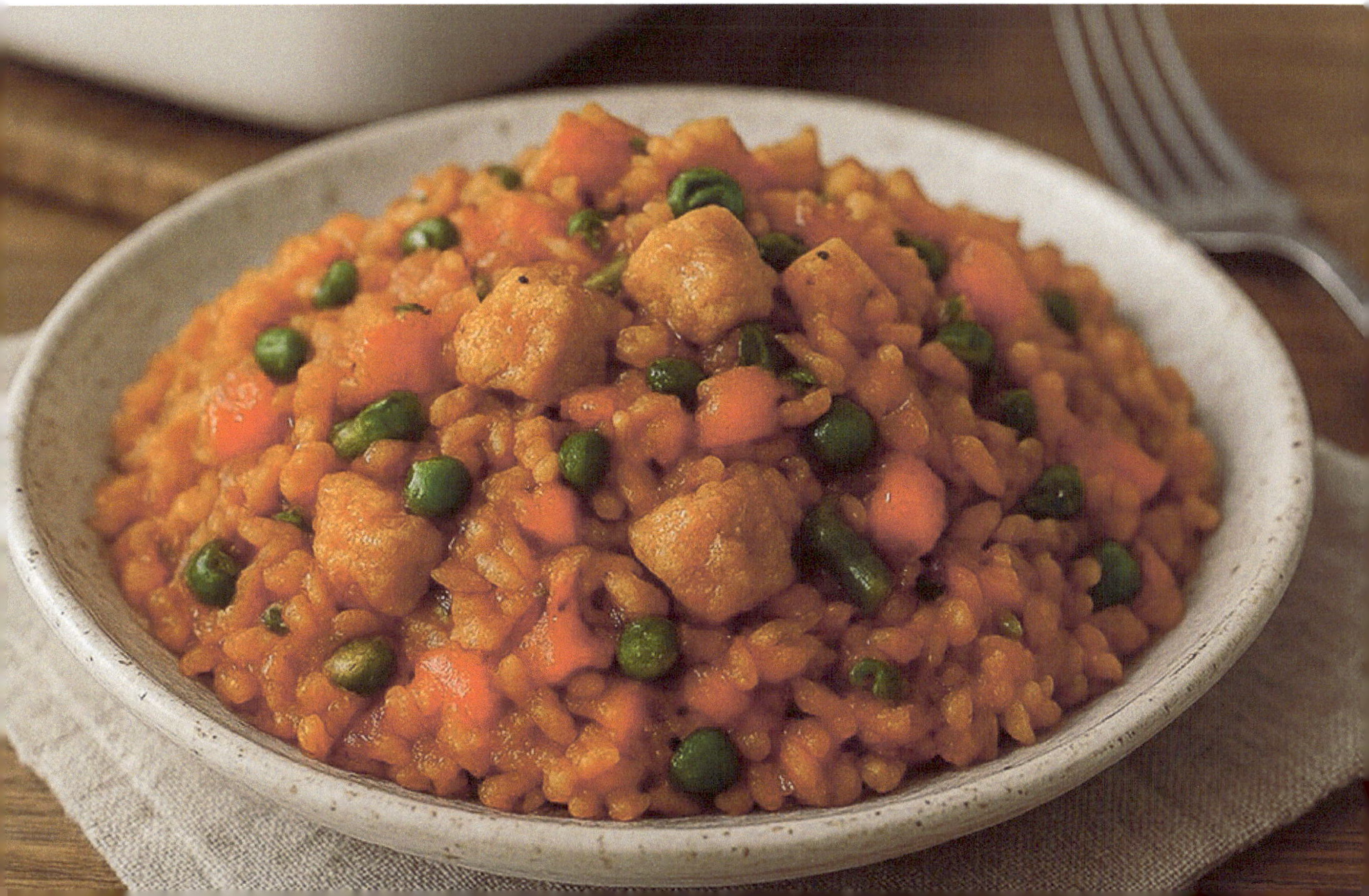

Healing Chicken Noodle Casserole

This dish is easy to throw together but is a complete meal that is soothing and warm.

Time

50 minutes total

Prep: 5 minutes

Bake: 45 minutes

Servings

8 servings

Tools

9" x 13" baking dish (or 2 8" x 8" pans or 2 9" round pans)

Ingredients

1/2 package egg noodles [227 g]

3 cans chicken (or 1 pound Tender Pot Chicken, prepared) [426 g]

2 cups frozen chopped veggies [270 g]

1 bouillon cube [4 g]

1 can cream of chicken condensed soup [312 g]

1 cup milk [227 g]

2 cups water [454 g]

1 teaspoon salt [6 g]

1/4 teaspoon oregano [1 g]

Directions

1. Preheat oven to 375. Mix all ingredients in a casserole dish. Bake for 45 minutes. Enjoy!

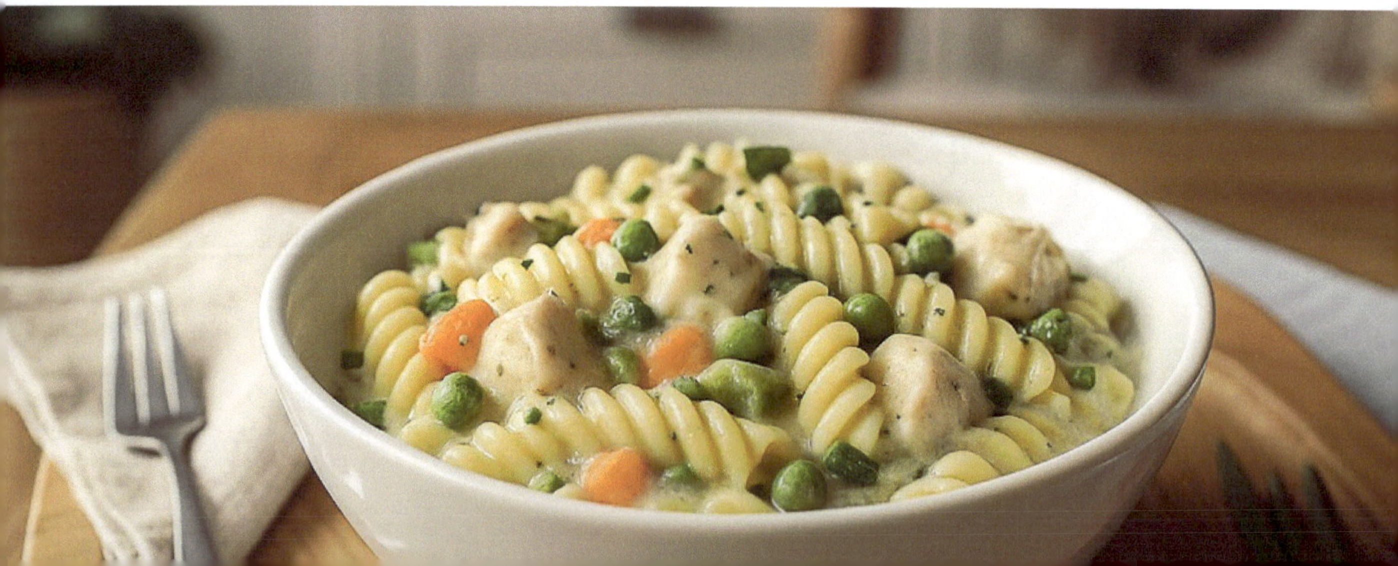

Creamy Broccoli Soup

Quick to make and delicious with a crusty sourdough bread!

Time

30 minutes

Servings

6 servings

Tools

2 medium pots

Spoon and/or ladle

Blender or immersion blender

Ingredients

1 package of frozen broccoli [340 g]

2 cups broth [240 g]

1 bay leaf

1/4 cup butter [56 g]

1/4 cup flour [30 g]

1 teaspoon salt [6 g]

1/4 teaspoon ground black pepper, or more to taste [1 g]

1 cup heavy whipping cream [240 g]

Directions

1. Put **1 package broccoli** into a medium pot with **2 cups broth** and **1 bay leaf**. Cook over high heat until the broccoli is bright green and fork tender.
2. While the broccoli is cooking, make a roux: melt **1/4 cup butter, then stir in 1/4 cup flour, 1 teaspoon salt,** and **1/4 teaspoon pepper**. Cook for one minute, stirring, then remove from heat.
3. Remove the bay leaf from the broccoli and broth, then blend the broccoli until it is a chunky puree (carefully transfer the hot soup into a blender, or leave it in the pot and use an immersion blender, careful not to splatter the hot liquid).
4. Pour the roux into the soup and stir to combine. Bring to a boil over medium-high heat, stirring occasionally.
5. Remove from heat and stir in **1 cup cream**. Serve hot.

Italian Greens Risotto

This is a delicious way to get your greens and will quickly become a comfort food for you. The chard must be fresh, but it can be rainbow chard (my favorite) or any kind of chard. Local chard grown in the cool months of early spring or late fall will taste the best. If the only chard you can get is bitter, you can parboil the chard prior to making the recipe; when you discard the boiling water, you will also be discarding the bitterness.

Time

20 minutes

Servings

4 servings

Tools

Knife

Cutting board

Medium pot

Large spoon

Small pan

Small spoon

Ingredients

1 bunch of Swiss chard

2 Tablespoons organic extra-virgin olive oil [26 g]

1/2 cup arborio rice [100 g]

2 cups broth (I enjoy chicken broth but have also made a delicious version with veggie bouillon and water. Add more broth for a soupier dish.) [480 g]

1 teaspoon salt [6 g]

1 Tablespoon butter [14 g]

1/4 cup pine nuts [36 g]

Parmesan cheese for topping (optional)

Directions

1. Wash **1 bunch of Swiss chard**. Remove stems and dice them.
2. Heat **2 Tablespoons olive oil** in a pot over medium-low heat. Add chard stems and **1/2 cup arborio rice**, and stir to coat with olive oil. Allow to cook for 2-3 minutes.

3. Add **2 cups broth** and **1 teaspoon salt** to the pot of rice. Bring to a boil and then reduce to a simmer. Cover and simmer until rice is just cooked.
4. Meanwhile, chop Swiss chard leaves into 1" pieces.
5. Melt **1 Tablespoon butter** in a small saucepan. Add **1/4 cup pine nuts.**
6. Cook pine nuts over medium-low heat, stirring frequently, until they are golden brown. Pay close attention so that they do not get too dark. Remove from heat.
7. Once the rice is cooked, add the Swiss chard leaves. Stir, and allow the leaves to wilt.
8. Serve in a bowl, topped with toasted pine nuts. You can also sprinkle on some shredded **parmesan cheese**, if desired.

When I visited Florence, Italy, and ordered Minestrone, every single time, they brought me a soup of Swiss chard and arborio rice. It was surprising and unfamiliar, but it was also delicious! Prior to this, I had thought that I didn't like Swiss chard, which was a shame because it is a very health-giving leafy green. I have adapted that Italian Minestrone into a risotto that is both light and warming.

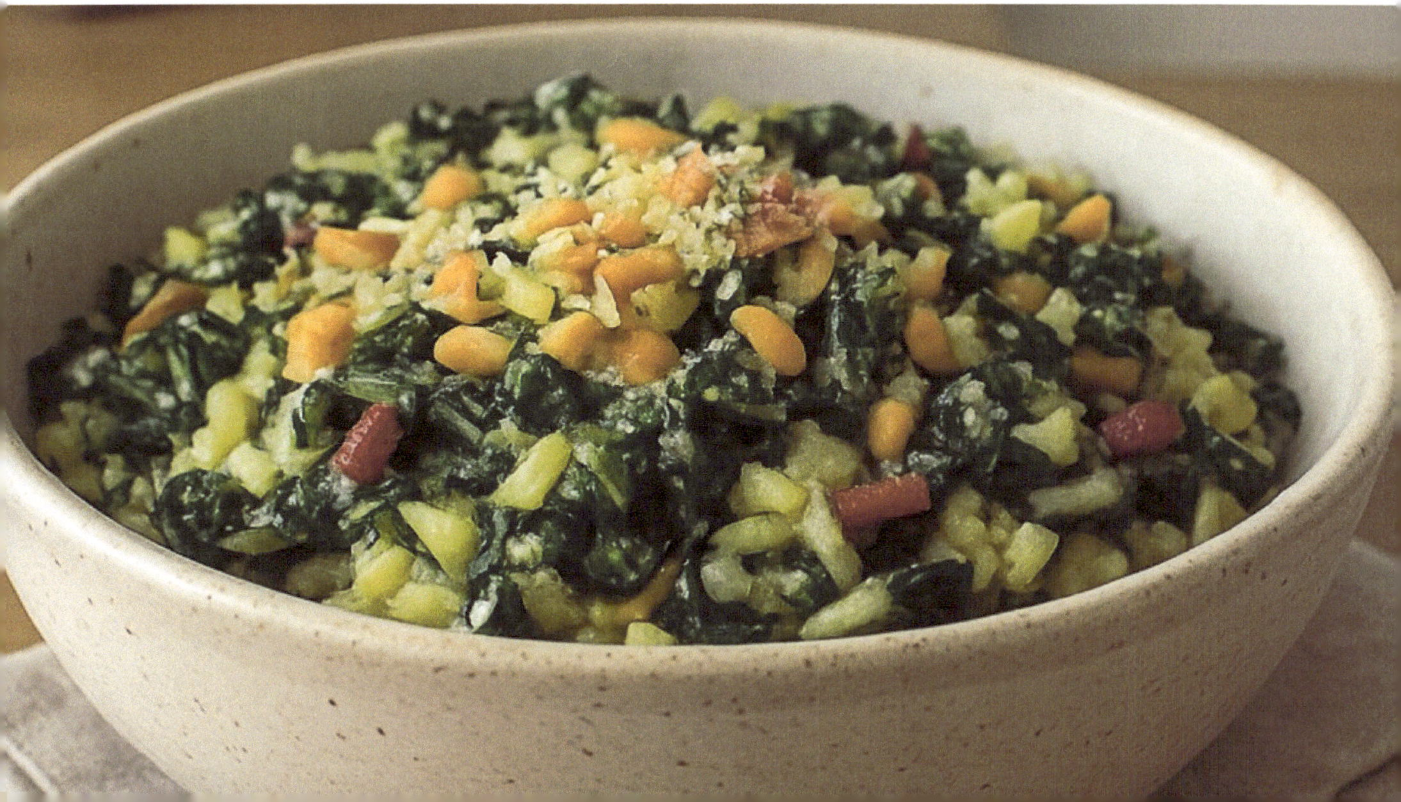

Easy One-Pot Clam Pasta

This recipe started as a healthier remake of a childhood favorite of mine: Pasta Roni Garlic Pasta. It has come a long way since then. Easy and delicious, it is a family favorite and quick to make with pantry staples. When you need to supercharge your immune system, the garlic in the recipe works well, but for other health reasons as discussed in the chapter on Food Choices, you may want to leave out the garlic cloves if you cannot source garlic scapes. It is delicious both with and without the garlic, and I appreciate that one ingredient can make this seem like two different recipes, adding variety to my repertoire.

Time

20 minutes

Servings

6 servings

Tools

Knife (optional)

Cutting board (optional)

Medium pot

Large spoon

Small pan

Small spoon

Ingredients

2 Tablespoons butter [28 g]

1-2 cloves garlic or 1-2 garlic scapes, diced (optional)

3 cups chicken broth [720 g]

1/2 teaspoon salt [3 g]

2 6.5-ounce cans of chopped clams [368 g]

1/2 pound angel hair pasta [227 g]

1 cup grated parmesan cheese [100 g]

1/2 cup heavy cream [120 g]

Parsley or oregano to taste for topping (optional)

Directions

1. In a pot, melt 2 Tablespoons butter.

2. While the butter is melting, dice **1-2 cloves garlic or 1-2 garlic scapes**, if you are including them, but don't let the butter brown.
3. Add the diced garlic or garlic scapes to the butter, if you are including them. Cook for 1-2 minutes over medium-low heat.
4. Add 3 cups chicken broth and 1/2 teaspoon salt.
5. Open **2 cans of clams**, and use the lids to strain the liquid into the pot; set the clams aside.
6. Raise the heat to high and bring to a boil.
7. Break **1/2 pound of angel hair pasta** into half or quarters (or smaller) and put it into the boiling liquid.
8. Cook the pasta for 4 minutes (or according to the package directions or your preference of softness).
9. Once the pasta is cooked, reduce the heat to low. Add a little bit of **parmesan cheese** at a time, stirring constantly, until you have added the full 1 cup. Continue stirring until it is completely melted.
10. Add the clams and **1/2 cup cream**. Stir until incorporated and warm.
11. Serve immediately, with **parsley or oregano** sprinkled on top, if desired.

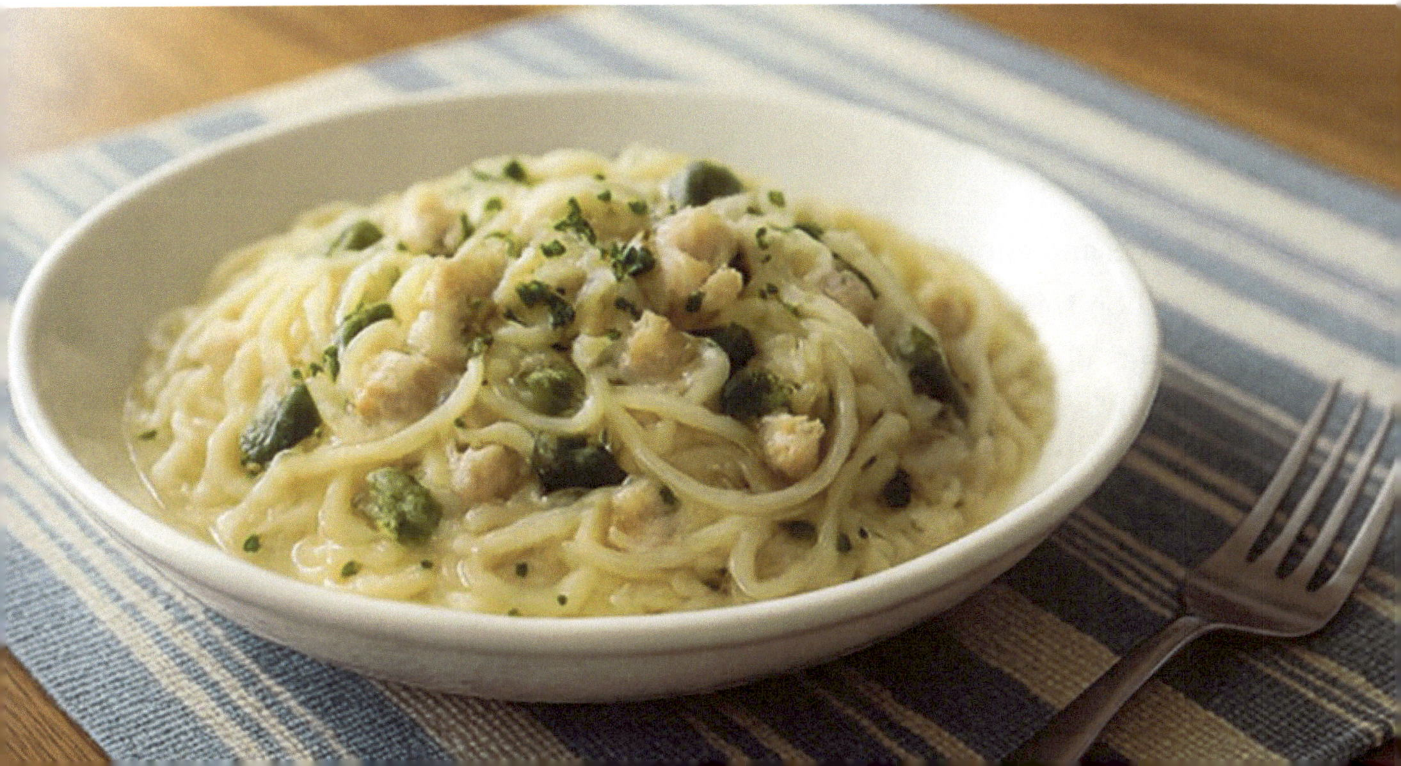

Swiss Chalet Potage

This smooth potato soup is mild and warming, especially nice served with crusty sourdough bread.

Time

30 minutes total

Prep: 10 minutes

Cook: 20 minutes

Servings

Approximately 2 servings

Tools

Knife

Potato peeler (optional)

Cutting board

Medium pot

Spoon

Immersion Blender

Ingredients

2 potatoes, peeled if you have the energy, and chopped

2 carrots, chopped

1/4 onion, chopped

1/4 cup of leafy greens or green beans, chopped

2 cups broth [480 g]

1/2 teaspoon salt [3 g]

Dash of paprika

Dash of black pepper

Directions

1. Peel and chop **2 potatoes** and **2 carrots**.
2. Chop **1/4 onion** and **1/4 cup leafy greens or green beans**.
3. Put all of those vegetables, plus **1/2 teaspoon salt**, a **dash of paprika**, a **dash of black pepper**, and **2 cups broth** into a pot and bring it to a boil over high heat.
4. Reduce the heat to low and simmer until all vegetables are soft.

5. Remove from heat and blend with an immersion blender until smooth.
6. Serve hot.

Why is this called Swiss Chalet Potage? On a ski trip with friends in the Swiss Alps, we were unexpectedly caught on the slopes in a terrifying, vicious blizzard. We clung desperately to the ski lift as it carried us, 100 feet above the ground, through wild winds and dashing, blinding snow. When we made it alive to the shelter of the ski chalet at the top of the slope, we were stunned, exhausted, and shivering. The proprietors didn't speak our language, but they knew to bring us big mugs of pale ale and steaming bowls of potato soup, which they called potage. It was the most hearty, warming, and comforting food we had ever tasted. No matter what challenge you are going through now, this potage will hearten you.

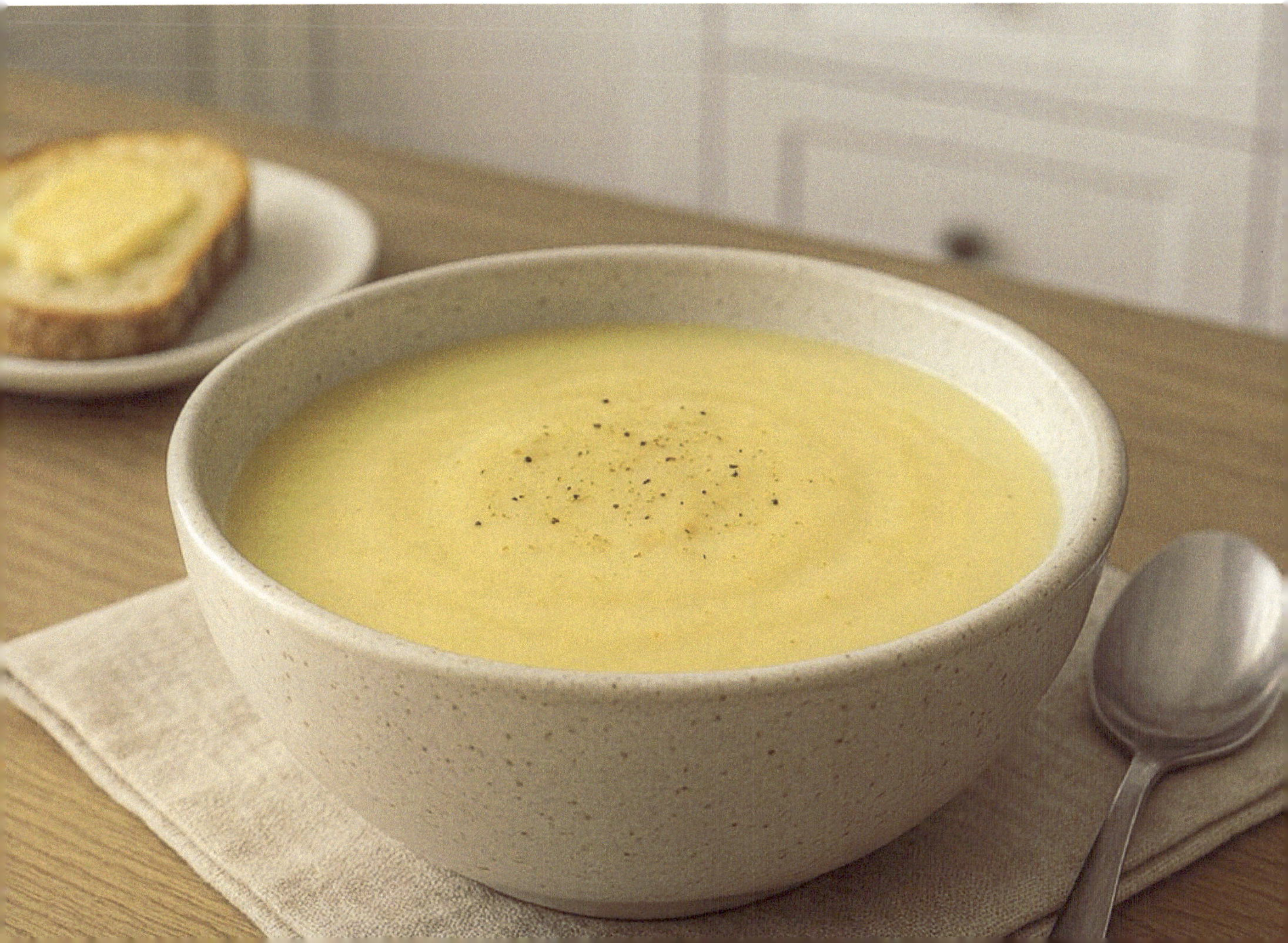

Warm Rice Porridge

My friend Shawchyi taught me this dish, and my Ayurveda practitioner and acupuncturist both encouraged me to choose porridge whenever I was feeling that my digestion was weak. Warm food cooked to softness is easy to digest, and you will be able to absorb nutrients and calories from it easily.

This recipe is a perfect way to make use of leftover rice, meat or vegetable dishes. Even when using leftovers, I often add frozen carrots and peas. If you have histamine issues, always pop your leftovers into the freezer as soon as your meal has ended; then, when you use leftovers for this dish, they will come out of the freezer in good condition for you.

Time

15 minutes total

Prep: 5 minutes

Cook: 10 minutes

Servings

1 serving

Tools

Small pot

Spoon

Ingredients

Rice (Chinese or Japanese rice, fresh or leftover (not brown or wild rice))

Steamed, roasted, or sautéed vegetables, cut into small pieces (leftover, fresh, or frozen)

Cooked meat, if desired, cut into small pieces

Broth (chicken or pork, preferred)

Splash of soy sauce

Salt to taste

Ginger, turmeric, garlic, basil, or any spices desired (optional)

Water, if needed

Directions

1. Put **rice, vegetables,** and **meat** into a pot, seasoning with soy **sauce, salt**, and your favorite **spices** but keeping the flavor mild.

2. Warm thoroughly over medium-low heat, stirring frequently, and adding **water** if needed to make it moist.
3. All ingredients should become soft and sticky.
4. Serve warm.

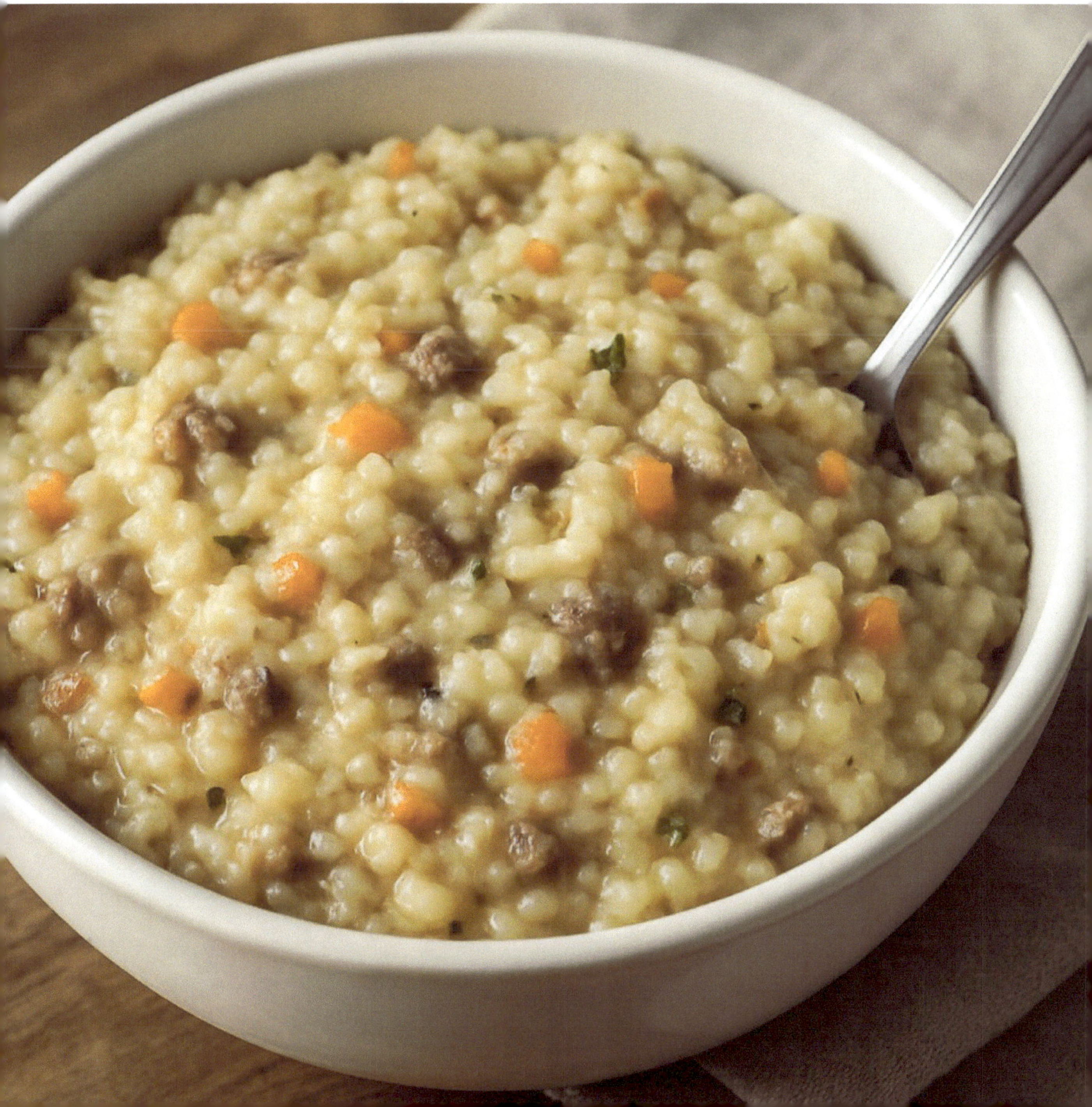

Simple Summer Pasta

The highlight of this dish is the fresh summer vegetables, but the benefit of making it is how little cooking it requires. Your kitchen will stay cool. Add whatever vegetables are in season that you would like to try.

Time

15 minutes

Servings

4 servings

Tools

Medium pot

Knife

Cutting board

Large bowl

Ingredients

8 ounces corkscrew pasta [227 g]

1 pint of cherry tomatoes (or other tomatoes) [300 g]

1/4 cup olive oil [50 g]

2 Tablespoons fresh basil, chopped (or other herb) [5 g]

3/4 teaspoon salt [4.5 g]

Shredded parmesan for topping, if desired

Directions

1. Prepare **8 ounces pasta** according to package directions.
2. While pasta is cooking, dice **1 pint tomatoes** and cut **2 Tablespoons basil leaves** into 1/4"-size pieces.
3. Put them into a large bowl. Add **1/4 cup olive oil, 3/4 teaspoon salt,** and cooked pasta, and stir to combine. Serve warm or cold, topped with parmesan.

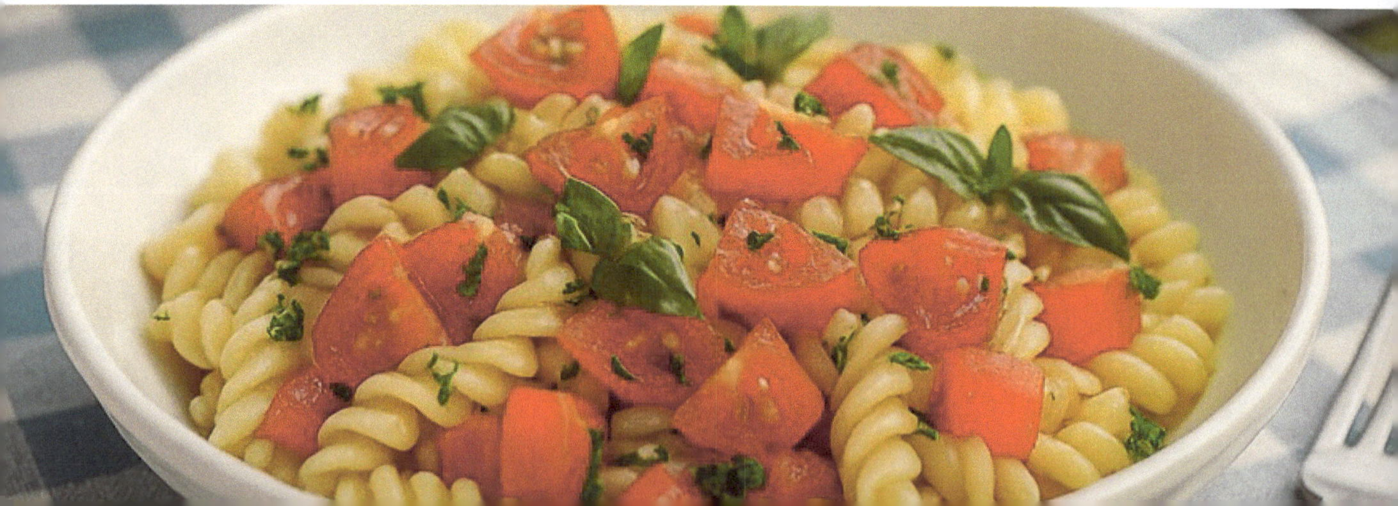

Potatoes and Eggs Comfort Skillet

This is a dish from my childhood. Although the ingredients would make it seem like breakfast, my family has always served it in the evening.

Time

30 minutes

Servings

4 servings

Tools

Knife

Cutting board

Skillet

Spatula

Ingredients

1/2 cup fat, bacon grease preferred [90 g]

4 potatoes

4 eggs

Salt to taste

Directions

1. Slice **4 potatoes** as thin as possible.
2. Melt **1/2 cup fat** in pan over medium-high heat.
3. Add potatoes to pan in flat layers. Leave the potatoes to cook until the ones on the bottom have begun to get crispy. Flip the potatoes and repeat.
4. Stir and flip the potatoes until they are all soft and as crispy as you can get them.
5. Turn the heat off but leave the pan on the hot stove (or turn the heat to low). Break **4 eggs** into the potatoes. Mix the potatoes until the eggs have all cooked, clinging to the potatoes.
6. **Salt** generously and serve.

Sheet Pan Wild Herb Gnocchi

When you need a really easy dinner, use pesto from a jar, but when the weather allows, choose wild herbs to make your own pesto. These herbs are mast cell stabilizers, anti-inflammatory, and have the nutrients that you specifically need to heal and get through crisis as quickly as possible. If wild herbs are not available, use fresh basil.

Time

25 minutes total

Active: 15 minutes

Bake: 10 minutes

Servings

6 servings

Tools

Knife

Cutting board

Casserole dish or rimmed baking sheet

Small pan

Spoon

Blender or immersion blender with jar

Mixing or serving bowl

Large spoon

Ingredients

1 package gnocchi (shelf stable or frozen) [420 g]

1 pound kielbasa sausage, sliced into bite-size rounds [454 g]

1 package frozen chopped broccoli [340 g]

Wild Herb Pesto Sauce:

- 2 Tablespoons butter [28 g]
- 1/4 cup pine nuts [36 g]
- 1 cup fresh wild herbs, washed and thick stems removed (Creeping Charlie or Purple Deadnettle, preferred) [20 g]
- 1/2 cup shredded parmesan cheese [50 g]
- 1/3 cup olive oil [67 g]

Directions

1. Preheat oven to 400 degrees. Pour all contents of **1 package gnocchi, 1 pound kielbasa cut into pieces**, and **1 package broccoli** into a casserole dish or rimmed baking sheet.
2. Bake for 15 minutes.
3. While the gnocchi is baking, prepare the Wild Herb Pesto Sauce: Melt **2 Tablespoons butter** in a small sauce pan over medium-low heat.
4. Add in **1/4 cup pine nuts**, and cook, stirring frequently, until pine nuts are golden brown. Allow to cool.
5. Place **1/2 cup shredded parmesan cheese, 1 cup herbs, 1/3 cup olive oil**, and cooled pine nuts into a blender or jar for use with an immersion blender.
6. When broccoli is just beginning to brown on the edges, remove gnocchi from oven, and transfer to a bowl.
7. Pour on pesto and stir to combine.
8. Serve hot.

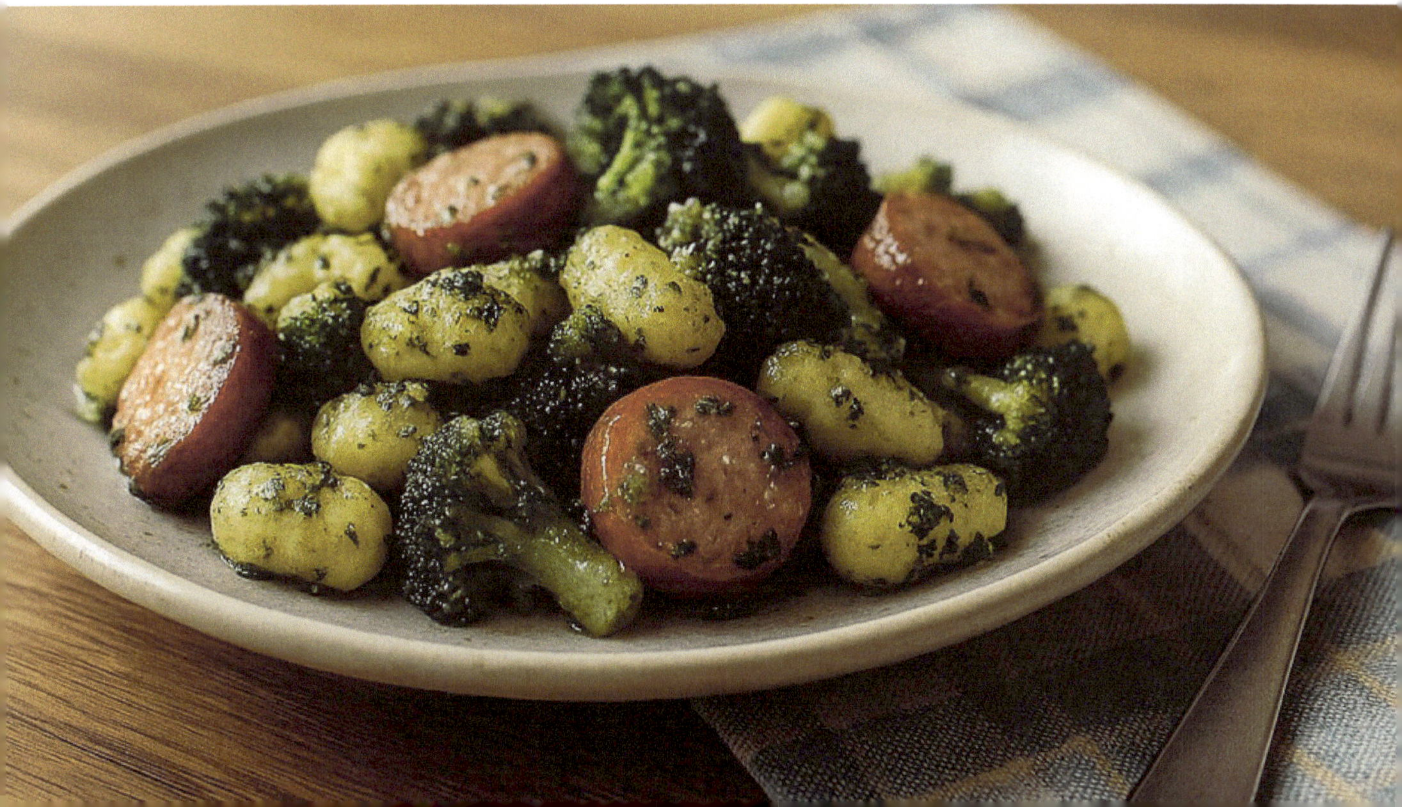

Greek Salmon Bowl

This meal has very robust flavor for surprisingly little effort. It is elegant with all of the toppings listed below, but it is perfectly satisfying with just kalamata olives and feta cheese, for days when the other toppings are too much work. I often serve this with leftover rice by adding a little bit of water to the rice and heating it on the stove, stirring occasionally until it is refreshed. Be aware that vinegar may be high histamine, so leave it out if your "histamine bucket" is full.

Time

15-30 minutes total

Active: 15 minutes

Cook: 15 minutes

Servings

1-2 servings

Tools

Small or medium pot with lid

Knife (optional)

Cutting board (optional)

Skillet

Spatula

Ingredients

1 filet of salmon (fresh or frozen, with or without skin) [115 g]

2 Tablespoons butter [28 g]

1 cup of warm cooked rice [200 g]

Toppings (optional):

- Kalamata olives
- Red onion, diced
- Fresh tomatoes, diced
- Feta cheese, crumbled
- Pine nuts (toasted or raw)

Simplest Greek Dressing:

- 1 Tablespoon balsamic vinegar [16 g]
- 1 Tablespoon olive oil [13 g]
- 1/2 Tablespoon real maple syrup (optional) [10 g]
- Salt and pepper to taste

Directions

1. Prepare rice according to package directions to make **1 cup cooked rice**.
2. Dry **1 salmon filet** with paper towel. **Salt** one or both sides of the salmon.
3. Melt **2 Tablespoons butter** in pan on medium heat.
4. Place salmon filet in butter, and cook about 5 minutes, until the bottom has become crispy and the salmon is cooked at least halfway through.
5. Flip the salmon, and cook it another few minutes until it is cooked through. You can cut into it to determine if it is done.
6. While salmon is cooking, prepare the Simplest Greek Dressing. Pour **1 Tablespoon vinegar, 1 Tablespoon olive oil**, and **1/2 Tablespoon syrup** into a jar, season with **salt** and **pepper** to taste.
7. Put a lid on the jar and shake.
8. Also prepare the toppings of your choice.
9. Spoon warm rice into a bowl, place salmon on top, and then sprinkle with your preferred toppings. Drizzle with dressing.

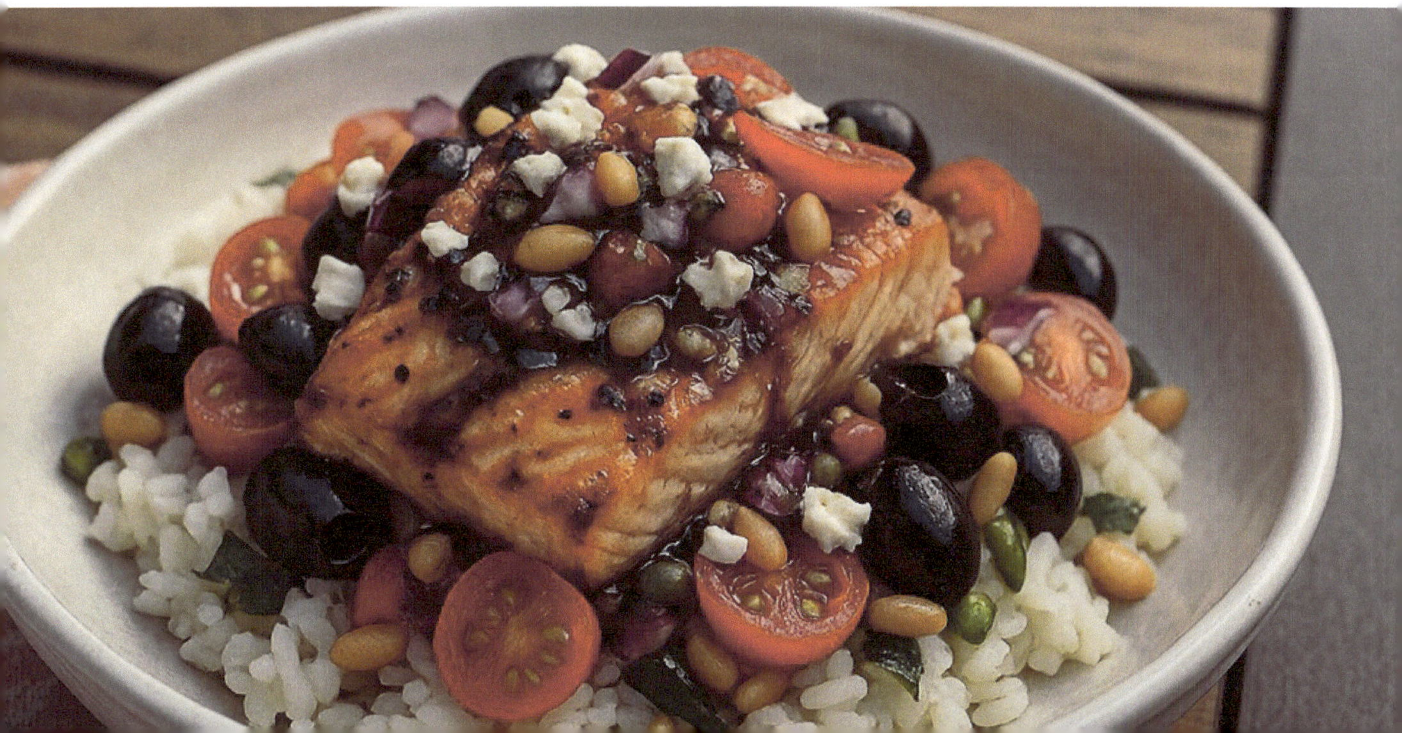

Wild and Wonderful Rice

Mix it up and let it cook. This is a safe meal for sensitive stomachs and pairs well as a side dish for chicken, pork, or fish.

Time

2 hours 10 minutes total

Prep: 10 minutes

Bake: 2 hours

Servings

4 servings

Tools

Knife

Cutting board

9” x 13” baking dish (or 2 8” x 8“ pans or 2 9” round pans)

Ingredients

2 carrots, diced

2 sticks of celery, diced

1 cup wild rice [160 g]

2 cups broth [480 g]

2 Tablespoons butter [28 g]

2 teaspoons salt [12 g]

Directions

1. Preheat oven to 300 degrees. Chop **2 carrots** and **2 sticks of celery**.
2. Mix carrots, celery, **1 cup wild rice, 2 cups broth, 2 Tablespoons butter,** and **2 teaspoons salt** in a casserole dish.
3. Bake for 2 hours.
4. Serve warm.

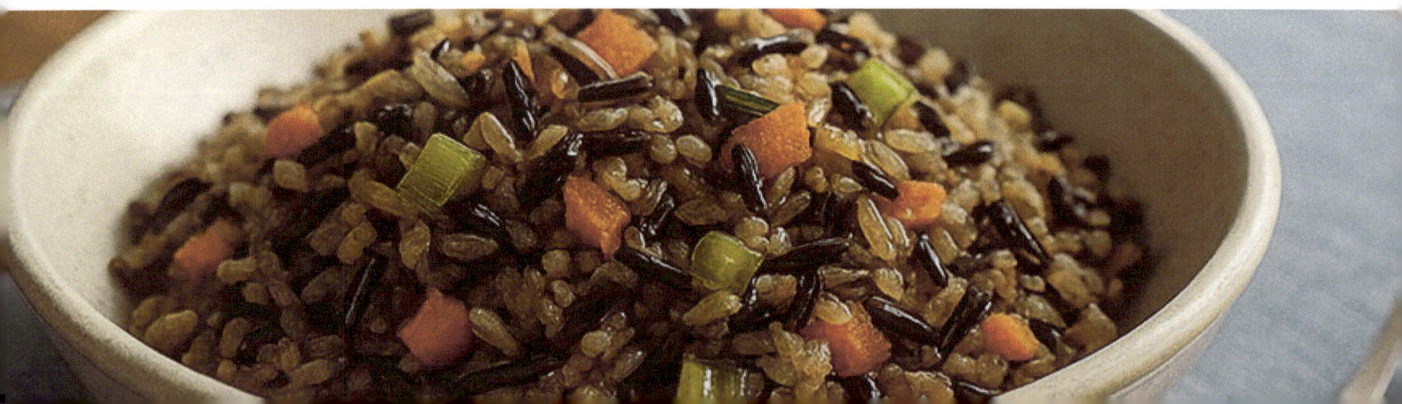

Easy Pot Roast Stew

This is a big hearty meal, but it is very easy to prepare. You will want to freeze some of it in single-serving bowls for the future. It turns out best in the Dutch oven, but using a slow cooker allows you to put it outside to cook so that the long-lasting cooking smell doesn't spark an MCAS episode.

Time

2-8 hours and 5 minutes total

Prep: 5 minutes

Cook: 2—8 hours

Servings

4 servings

Tools

Knife

Cutting board

Slow cooker or Dutch oven with lid

Spatula

Ingredients

1 beef roast (chuck, brisket, or bottom round, frozen or thawed)

2 carrots or 1 package baby carrots

1 onion, peeled and cut into quarters

2 potatoes, chopped into large bite-size pieces

1 cup broth [240 g]

Salt and pepper to taste

Directions

1. Place all ingredients into a Dutch oven or slow cooker (meat in first and veggies on top), and cook on low heat until it is soft. If using a Dutch oven with lid, set the oven to 350 degrees and cook approximately 2 hours. If using the slow cooker, choose the low setting and cook 8 hours.

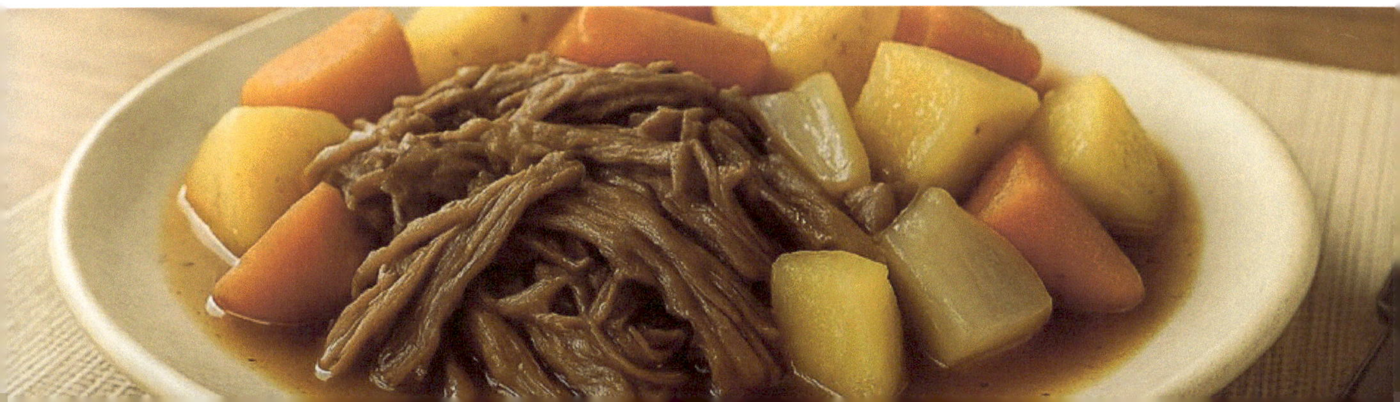

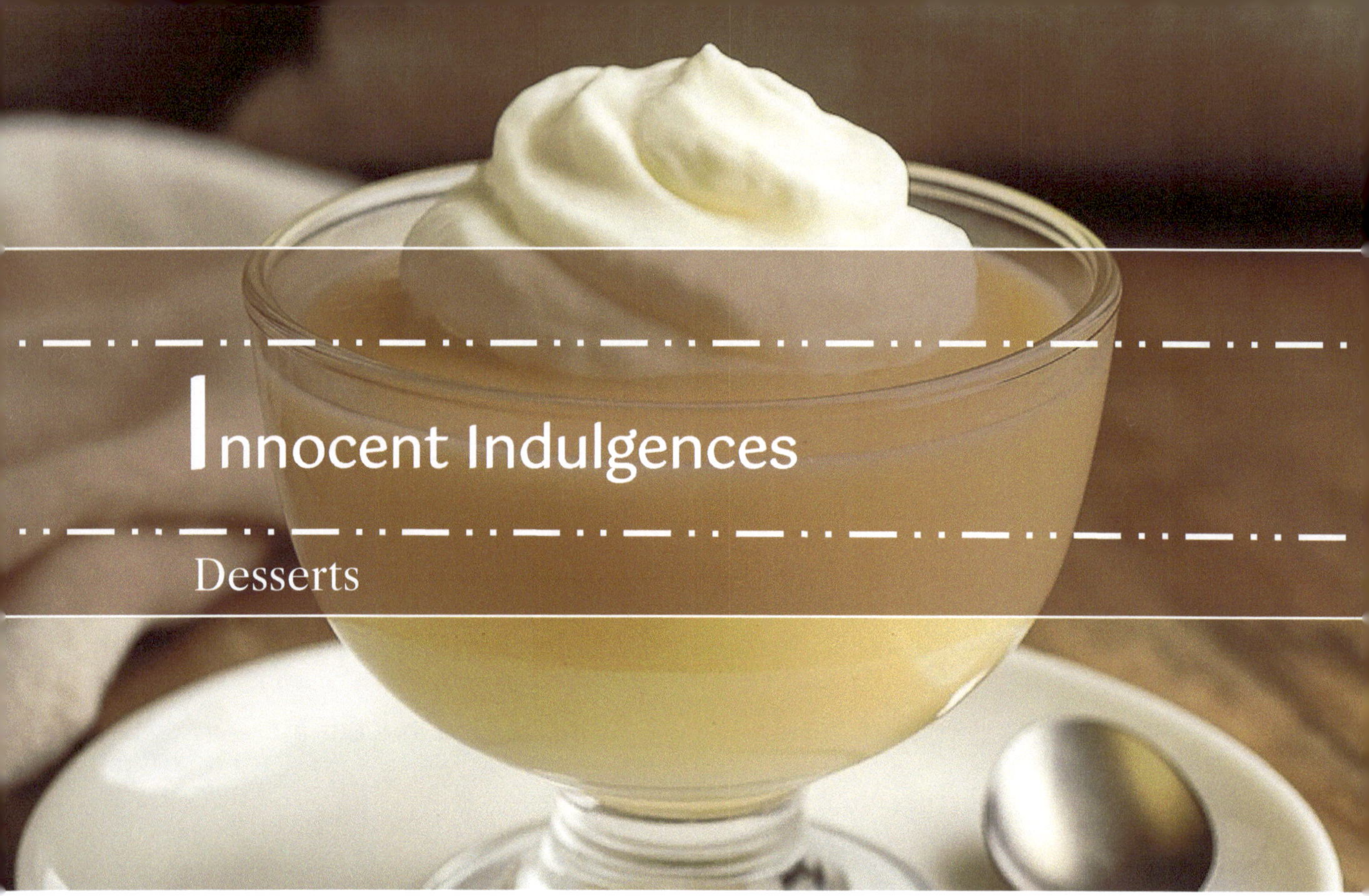

Innocent Indulgences

Desserts

Rich Maple Pudding

This is a comfort food that is easy on the stomach and so much healthier and tastier than box-mix or store-bought options. The hardest part is the stirring, so use a battery-powered pot stirrer, or pull up your stool to the stovetop and prepare for meditative cooking.

Time

15-30 minutes

Active: 10 minutes

Cooling: 5-20 minutes

Servings

4 servings

Tools

Medium pot

Whisk or spoon

Ingredients

3 Tablespoons cornstarch [30 g]

1/2 teaspoon salt [3 g]

1/3 cup real maple syrup [104 g]

2 cups raw whole milk [454 g]

1 teaspoon vanilla extract [4 g]

Whipped cream for topping (optional)

Directions

1. Using a whisk, mix **3 Tablespoons cornstarch** and **1/2 teaspoon salt** in a small pot.
2. Add **1/3 cup syrup** and **2 cups milk**. Whisk until well combined.
3. Heat pot over medium heat, stirring constantly with a whisk, until mixture comes to a soft boil, about 8 minutes.
4. Remove pot from heat and stir in **1 teaspoon vanilla**.
5. Allow pudding to cool until it reaches the desired thickness and temperature, stirring occasionally.
6. For the most delightful experience, serve warm with cold **whipped cream** on top. However, the pudding will also be good cooled or even chilled.

Berries with Cream

My grandmother taught me this dessert, which we sometimes enjoyed for breakfast. I find that modern people have forgotten some of the simplest traditional recipes that really highlight the flavor and health benefits of the ingredients the most. It is wonderful with freshly picked raspberries, but frozen raspberries are very good too – just thaw them for half an hour or so before using them.

Time

2 minutes

Servings

1 serving

Tools

Small dessert bowl

Ingredients

1/4 cup raspberries

2 Tablespoons heavy whipping cream [30 g]

Directions

1. Put **1/4 cup raspberries** into a small dessert bowl.
2. Pour **2 Tablespoons cream** over them.
3. Enjoy! You might like to crush some of the berries with your spoon before eating this.

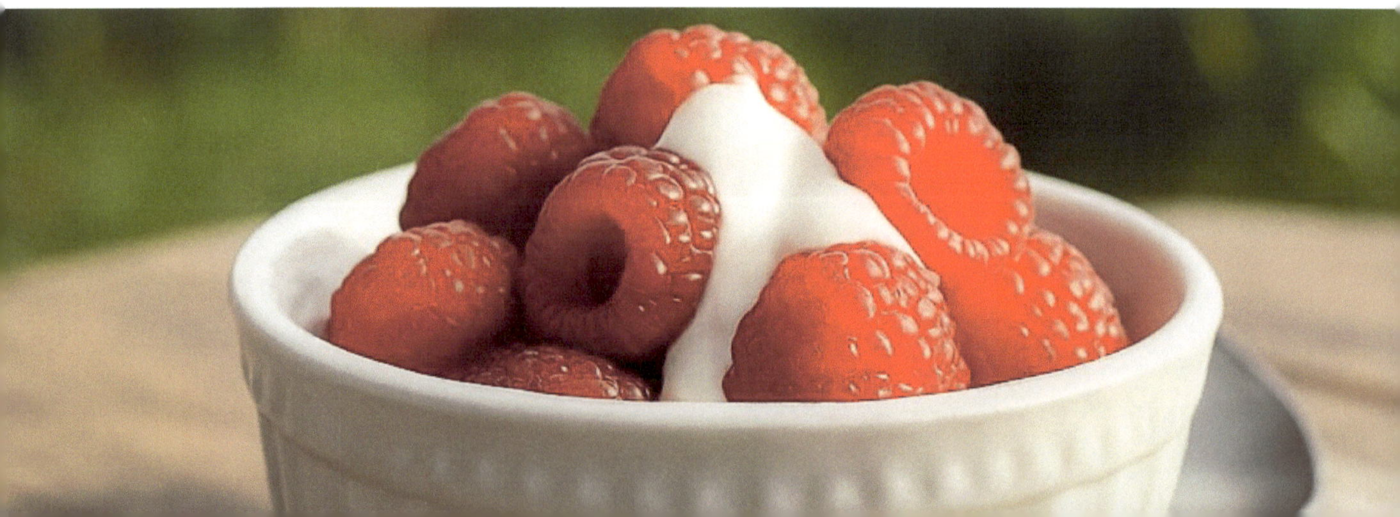

3-ingredient Cheesecake Strawberries

You deserve cheesecake when you are in crisis, but you also deserve not to have to make one! This recipe is as easy as can be. Storebought strawberries can be high in histamine, but local, fresh strawberries are full of nutrients.

Time

5 minutes

Servings

1 serving

Tools

Small sharp knife

Small bowl

Spoon

Ingredients

Fresh strawberries, washed and tops removed

1/4 cup cream cheese [57 g]

1 Tablespoon real maple syrup [20 g]

1 graham cracker, broken into approximately 1" pieces

Directions

1. Remove the tops of the **strawberries**, cutting a cone shape out of the top so that when the leaves are removed, there is a small bowl in the top of the berry.
2. Stir together **1/4 cup cream cheese** and **1 Tablespoon syrup**.
3. Place a dollop of the sweetened cheese on top of a strawberry.
4. Plunk a piece of **graham cracker** into the cheese dollop, and then pop the entire treat into your mouth.

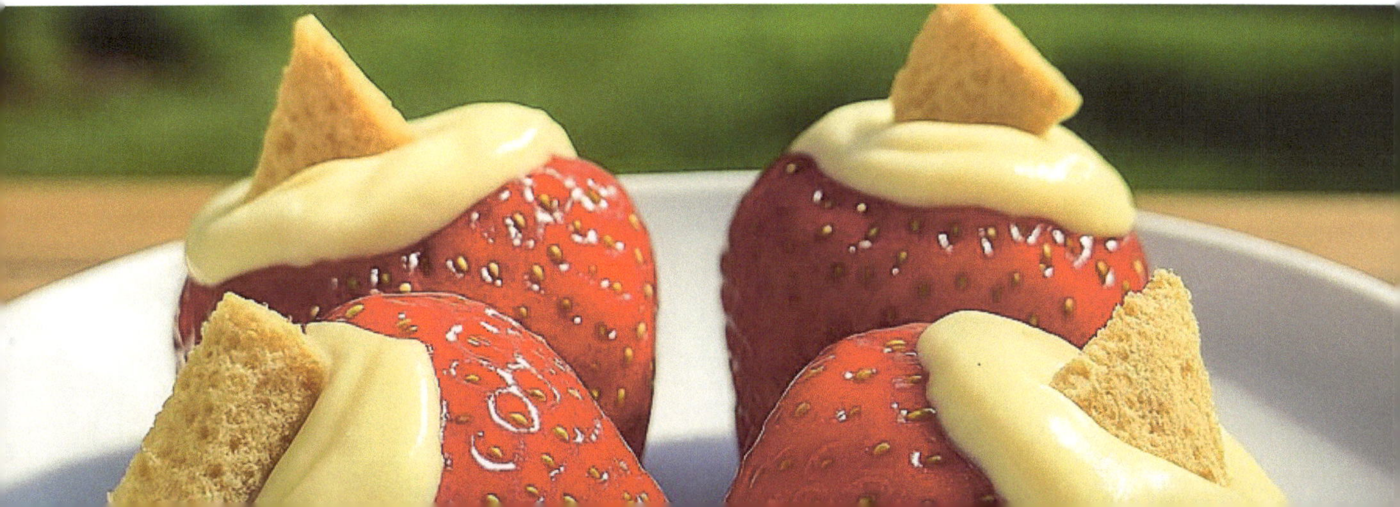

Dad's Freezie Fruit Salad

Dad invented this salad, traditionally made with a can of fruit cocktail in sugar syrup and a fruit-on-the-bottom yogurt. Those options are even easier than my version, for days when you really don't have energy to do more.

Time

5-10 minutes

Servings

1 serving

Tools

Small bowl

Cover for bowl (such as plastic wrap or wax wrap)

Ingredients

1 cup fresh fruit, chopped (bananas, apples, oranges, strawberries, and blueberries)

1 Tablespoon jam or jelly (raspberry or cherry) [20 g]

2 Tablespoons plain whole-milk yogurt [30 g]

Directions

1. Mix **1 Tablespoon jam** and **2 Tablespoons yogurt** in a small bowl. (You can use the bowl you're going to eat out of if you're only making one serving.)
2. Add **1 cup chopped mixed fruit** and stir.
3. Cover with a plastic wrap or wax wrap.
4. Put the bowl of fruit salad into the freezer for 30 minutes. The yogurt should get a little slushy but not frozen.
5. Remove from the freezer, stir, and enjoy.

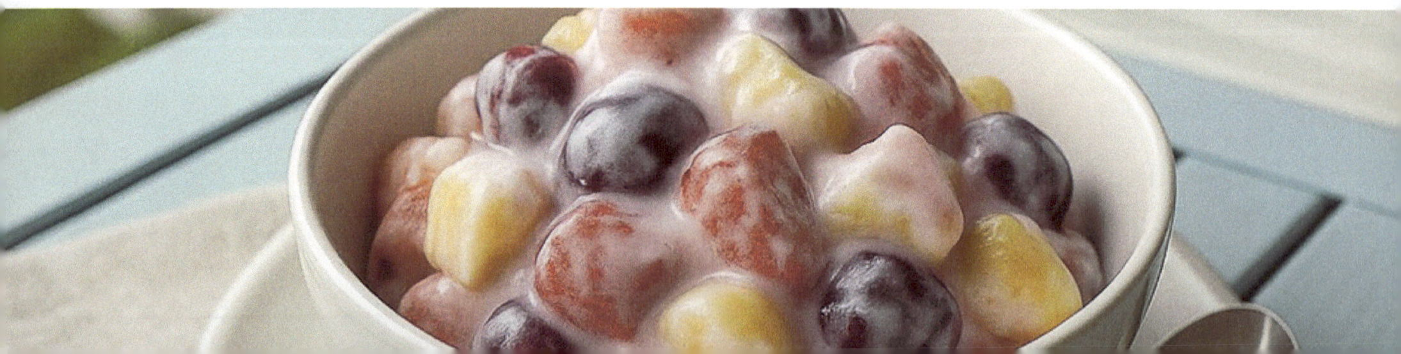

No-Bake Blueberry Tart

Naturally sweet, blueberries also have a magical quality of firming up like a gelatin dessert without any added ingredients!

Time

10 minutes

Servings

2 servings

Tools

Food processor

2 single-serving pie dishes or dessert bowls

Ingredients

1/4 cup pecans [27 g]

1/4 cup almonds [36 g]

1/4 teaspoon cinnamon (optional) [1 g]

1/2 teaspoon maple syrup or honey, adjusted [3 g]

1 cup fresh blueberries [148 g]

Whipped cream for topping, if desired

Directions

1. Put **1/4 cup pecans** and **1/4 cup almonds** into food processor and blend until finely ground.
2. Add **1/4 teaspoon cinnamon** and **1/2 teaspoon maple syrup**, and blend until well combined. The mixture will be dry but should stick together if pinched; if it does not stick together, add more syrup.
3. Press nut mixture into 2 single-serving pie dishes or dessert bowls.
4. Clean the bowl of the food processor. Put in **1 cup fresh blueberries** and blend until pureed.
5. Pour the blueberries into the piecrusts, and wait 10 minutes.
6. Serve immediately, with **whipped cream** on top if desired.

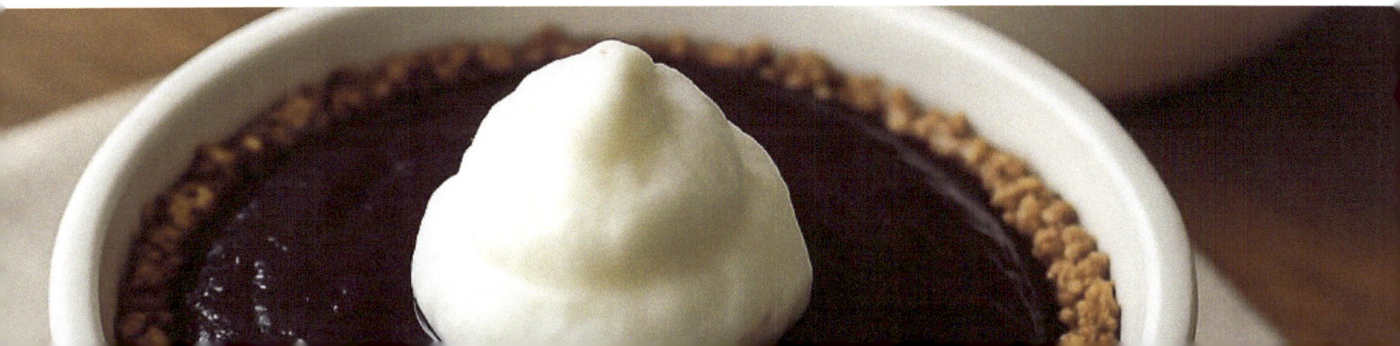

Healthy Chocolate Syrup

This Healthy Chocolate Syrup contains lots of beneficial nutrients and nothing bad. Use it on ice cream, for making chocolate milk, and in the 2-Ingredient Decadent Mousse. The water content allows it to stay liquid in the refrigerator, and it can be stored in a jar with a narrow spout and lid for many future easy uses. If you want a thicker, fudgier sauce, leave out the water and serve this Healthy Chocolate Syrup warm. Chocolate milk is a recommended after-workout recovery aid.

Time

10 minutes

Servings

8 servings

Tools

Pot

Whisk

Ingredients

1 cup maple syrup [312 g]

1/2 cup cocoa powder [42 g]

2 Tablespoons water [30 g]

Directions

1. Heat **1 cup maple syrup** in a medium pot over medium-high heat, stirring occasionally with a whisk.
2. When the syrup is warm, add **1/2 cup cocoa powder**, stirring continuously and scraping the sides until the cocoa powder is melted and incorporated.
3. Stir in **2 Tablespoons water**.

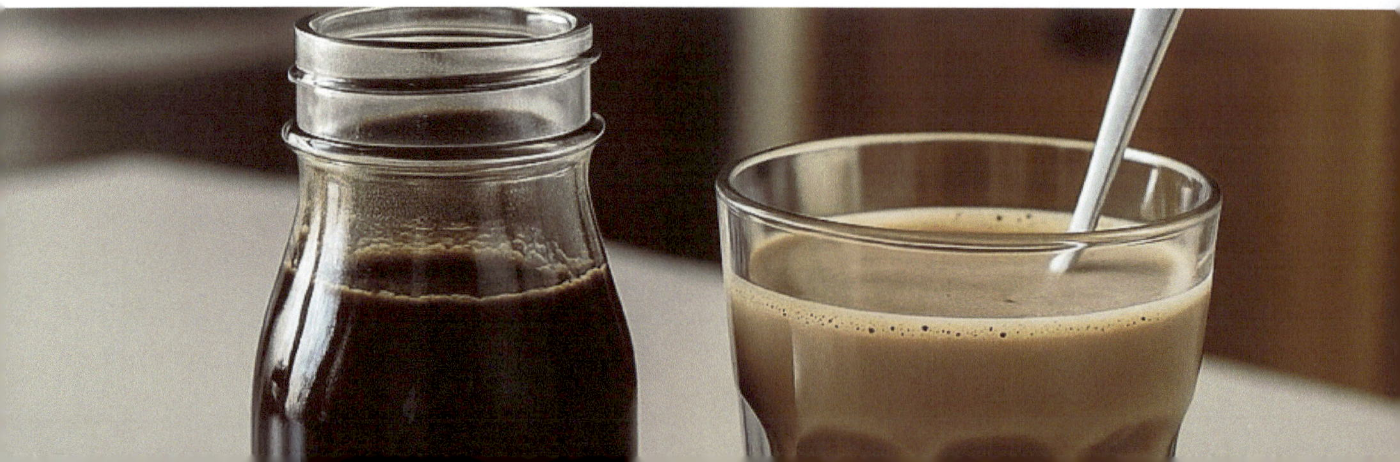

2-Ingredient Decadent Mousse

This is the fastest, easiest, fanciest dessert you'll ever make. You could also put it into the nut piecrusts from the No-Bake Blueberry Tart recipe for a simplified version of Chocolate French Silk Pie.

Time

10 minutes

Servings

2 servings

Tools

Mixing bowl or stand mixer with bowl

Whisk or whisk attachment for stand mixer

Ingredients

1 cup heavy whipping cream [227 g]

1 cup Healthy Chocolate Syrup, chilled (from previous recipe) [236 g]

Whipped cream for topping (optional)

Directions

1. Put **1 cup heavy whipping cream** into the bowl and whip on high speed until it begins to thicken. If whipped cream for topping is desired, you can make extra during this step, set it aside, and mix in sifted powdered sugar.
2. While continuing to whisk, drizzle in **1 cup Chocolate Syrup**.
3. Whisk until peaks form and the mousse has reached the desired consistency.
4. Serve immediately with **whipped cream**, if desired.

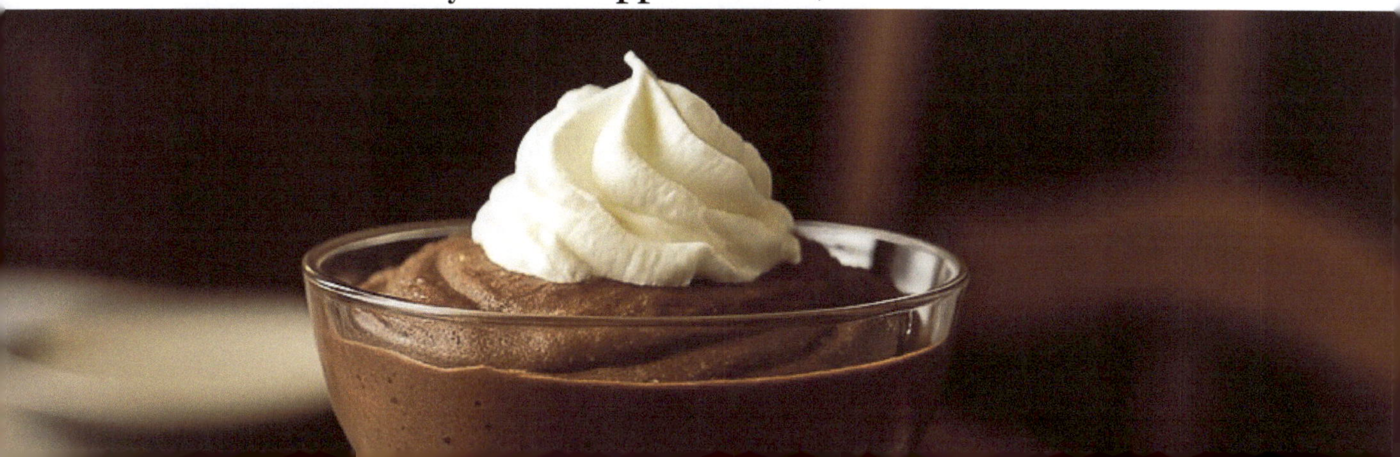

Garden Mint Ice Cream

Mint is very good for you and can help relieve congestion, nausea, and the common cold. It is also delicious and refreshing. Mint is usually very easy to grow or to find in a wilderness park, but you can also buy it in the produce section of the grocery store. An ice cream maker of some kind is necessary. This Garden Mint Ice Cream is a special treat with Healthy Chocolate Syrup (see the next recipe) drizzled over it!

Time

45 minutes total

Prep: 5-10 minutes

Freeze: 25 minutes (or whatever your ice cream maker requires)

Servings

8 servings

Tools

Jar, pot, or large mug

Tools for boiling 1 cup water

Strainer

Ice cream maker

Mixing bowl

Whisk or spoon

Ingredients

1 bunch fresh mint leaves, stems intact or removed

1 cup water, boiling [227 g]

1 cup raw whole milk [227 g]

1 cup heavy whipping cream [227 g]

3/4 cup real maple syrup [234 g]

1 teaspoon vanilla extract, alcohol-free preferred [4 g]

Directions

1. Place **1 bunch of mint leaves** in a jar, and pour **1 cup boiling water** over them.
2. Allow this mint tea to steep for 10 minutes.

3. Strain out the leaves, pouring the tea into a stand mixer bowl or regular mixing bowl.
4. Add **1 cup milk, 1 cup cream, ¾ cup syrup,** and **1 teaspoon vanilla,** and stir to combine.
5. Follow the directions for your ice cream maker with this mixture.

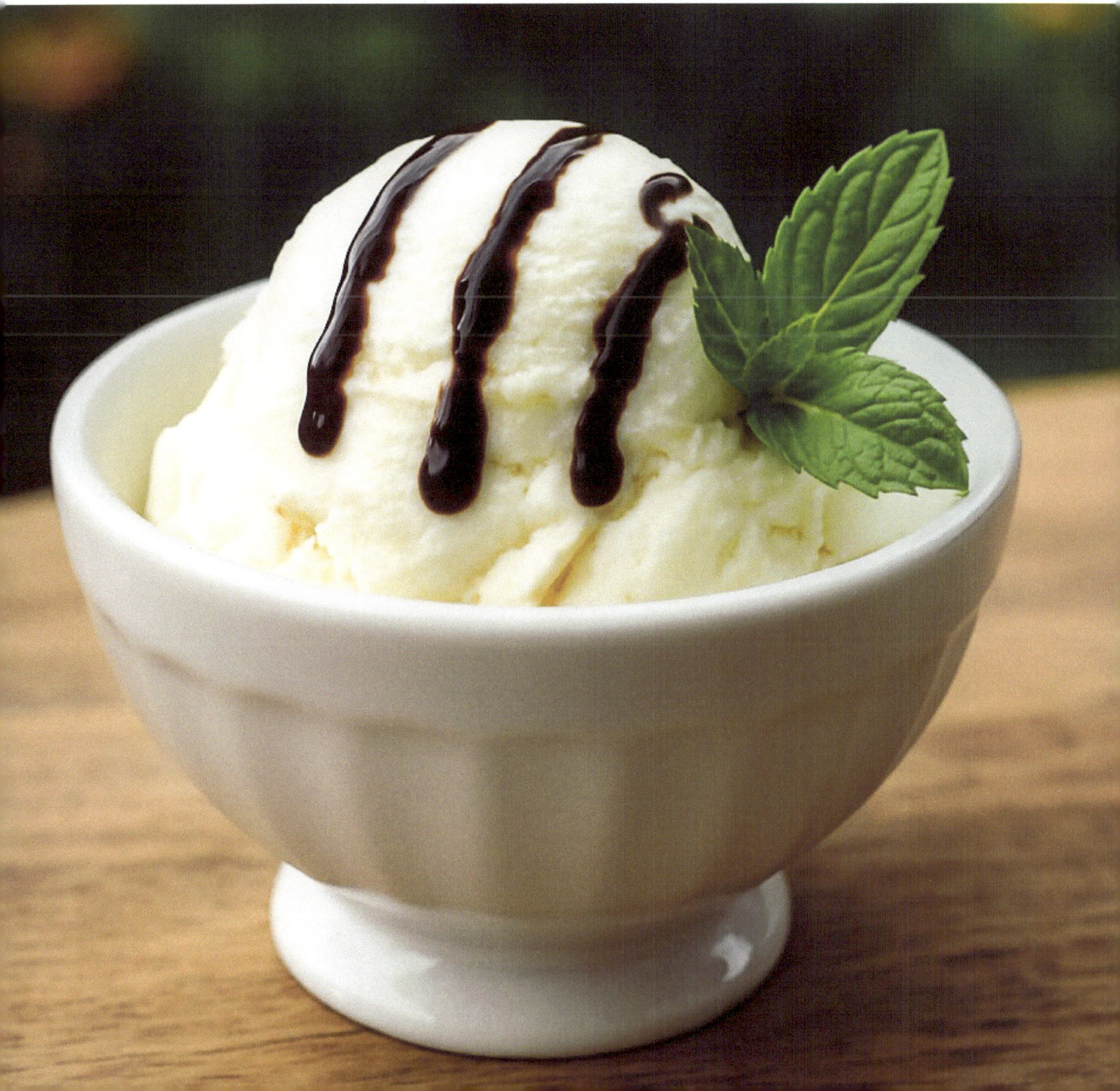

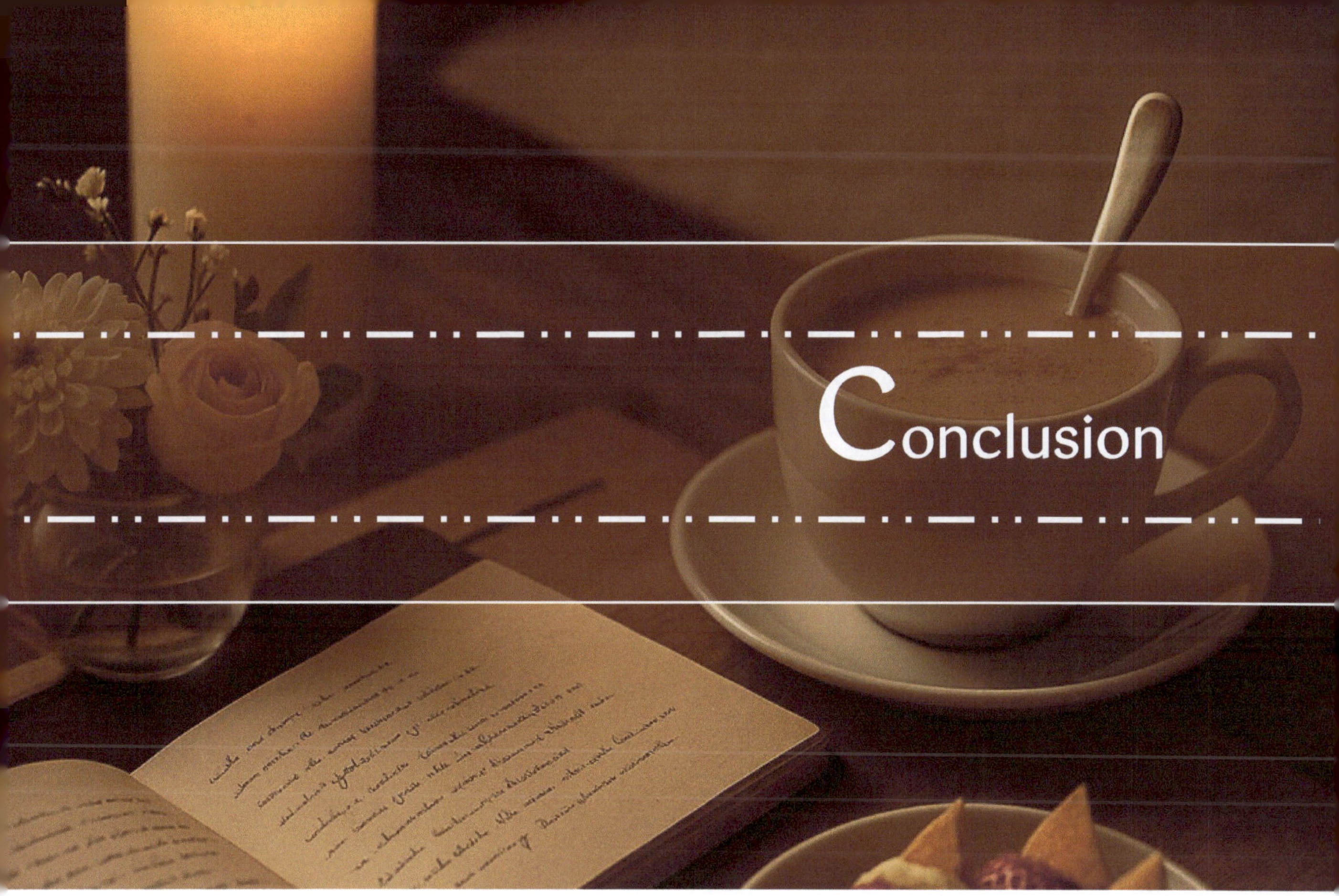

Conclusion

When I told my son the list of recipes that I was including in this book, he said, “But Mom, you’re leaving out all of your best recipes! What about your muffins? They’re the best muffins I’ve ever had!”

It is true, my best recipes are not my easiest recipes, but I think you’ll find these easy ones tastier than most of what you’ve been eating lately. Most importantly, this book has been designed to get you through hard times. And to help you heal.

Your body, your heart, and your spirit will, I hope, recover from your setbacks and move out of the season of crisis into a season of happiness and better health.

You may have setbacks again in the future, but with what you have learned this time, perhaps you will handle the difficulties more easily. Maybe the hard seasons will be shorter in the future. Maybe you will even learn how to glean benefits from the hard seasons, get more out of them, and come out even better than ever.

You are ready, now, for the best recipes. I have a few cookbook ideas in mind, as well as plans for other kinds of books...but the book I've been working on simultaneously with this one is tentatively titled *Cooking with Our Ancestors*. That book will contain a lot of my best recipes, along with channeled information about cooking traditions from across the ages and guidance on how to use cooking as a tool to harness and enhance your intuitive skills. Another cookbook I am working on will have my very best recipes, destined for your holiday tables and, as always, made with the most health-giving and delightful ingredients and love.

Please leave a review at the online store wherever you purchased this cookbook! Here are QR codes for the Amazon page and Good Reads:

About the Author

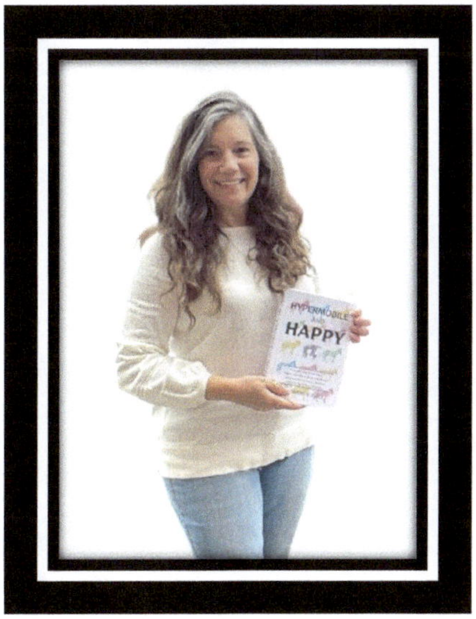

Shannon E. Gale has been named one of the **Top 20 Inspiring Women to Look For in 2025** by ***NY Weekly Magazine***, and she has been honored in ***Marquis' Who's Who***. Her 2024 book, *Hypermobile and Happy*, won an **International Impact Book Award** and has inspired a devoted international following on social media.

Shannon is a housewife and homeschooling mother. She spends most of her time cooking for her family, a blessing she thoroughly enjoys. Previously, Shannon has been the founder and director of the Vibrant Life holistic healing center, Gale Force Dance professional performance company, Circle Play and Learn Academy forest school, Frankfort School of Ballet studio, and Helpful Editor professional services. She enjoys walking in the woods, playing pickleball, reading novels, kayaking, and playing board games. She lives in Kentucky with her loving husband, delightful 12-year-old son, and senior "puppy" dog.

Find Shannon at **www.shannonegale.com** and on social media under her name or **@hypermobileandhappy**.

Index of Recipes

Everyday Nourishment (Main Dishes)

Innocent Indulgences (Desserts)

Index of Ingredients

www.ingramcontent.com/pod-product-compliance
Lightning Source LLC
LaVergne TN
LVHW070936210926
848482LV00003B/255
* 9 7 8 1 9 6 5 0 2 0 0 3 6 *